NATIONAL
HEALTH INSURANCE
in the United States and Canada

American Governance and Public Policy Series

Series Editors: Gerard W. Boychuk, Karen Mossberger, and Mark C. Rom

Historical Development of Public Health Insurance in the United States and Canada, 1910–60

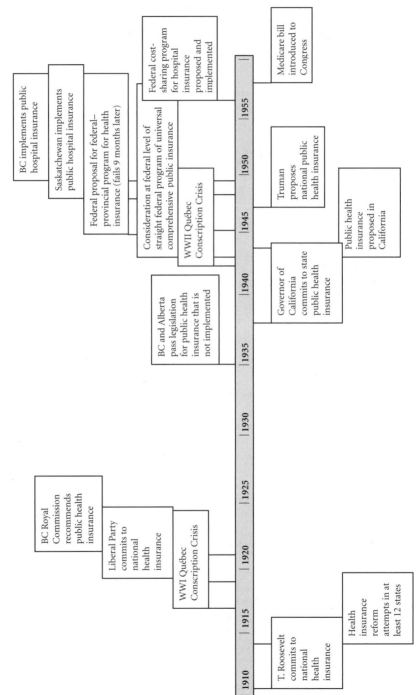

Historical Development of Public Health Insurance in the United States and Canada, 1960–2005

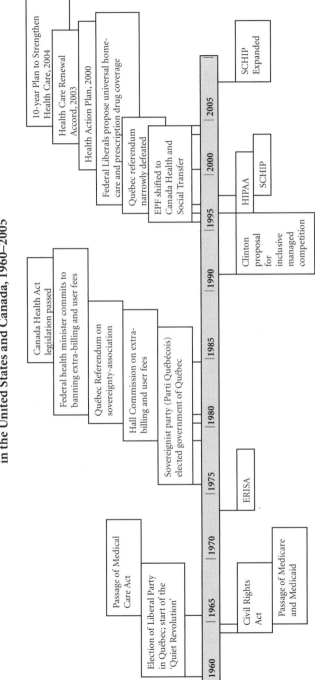

NATIONAL
HEALTH INSURANCE
in the United States and Canada

*Race, Territory, and
the Roots of Difference*

GERARD W. BOYCHUK

Georgetown University Press / Washington, D.C.

Georgetown University Press, Washington, D.C. www.press.georgetown.edu

Library of Congress Cataloging-in-Publication Data

Boychuk, Gerard William, 1967–
  National health insurance in the United States and Canada : race, territory, and the roots of difference / Gerard W. Boychuk.
      p.   ; cm. — (American governance and public policy series)
  Includes bibliographical references and index.
  ISBN 978–1-58901–206–6 (alk. paper)
  1. National health insurance—United States—History—20th century.   2. National health insurance—Canada—History—20th century.   I.   Title.   II. Series: American governance and public policy.
  [DNLM: 1. National Health Insurance, United States—history—Canada.
2. National Health Insurance, United States—history—United States.   3. History, 20th Century—Canada.   4. History, 20th Century—United States.   5. History, 21st Century—Canada.   6. History, 21st Century—United States.   7. Politics—Canada.
8. Politics—United States.   9. Race Relations—history—Canada.   10. Race Relations—history—United States.   11. Single-Payer System—history—Canada.
12. Single-Payer System—history—United States. W 275 AA1 B789n 2008]

RA412.2.B69   2008
368.4'2—dc22   2007045440

15 14 13 12 11 10 09 08   9 8 7 6 5 4 3 2
First printing

Printed in the United States of America

For Debora and ShanLin

CONTENTS

ILLUSTRATIONS

Tables

Figures

PREFACE

S PENDING A SABBATICAL YEAR in Ann Arbor and East Lansing, Michigan, and Durham, North Carolina, in 2005 powerfully reinforced my perceptions of the continuing pervasiveness of the issue of race in American politics. I became more and more convinced about an argument that I had been making to my students: if an American were to visit Canada and vice versa and each visitor was then asked to summarize in a single phrase the most distinctive aspect of the political and social system of the country they had just visited, the Canadian observer would likely point to the prevalence of the politics of race in the United States and the American observer would likely point to the territorial politics of language and region in Canada—especially the issue of Québec's place in the Canadian federation.

Given this, it is surprising that very few accounts of the development of health care policy in the United States pay adequate attention to the role of racial politics. In providing an overview of existing explanations of the lack of national health insurance in the United States, Jill Quadagno considers an explanation that "attributes the failure of national health insurance to the racial politics of the South" (2005, 13). She provides only a single citation (with no page number) to an example of this argument—Robert Lieberman's *Shifting the Color Line*. Surprisingly to readers following up Quadagno's reference, the index to Lieberman's book does not include a single reference to health insurance. The passage and citation are very revealing. One would expect—as Quadagno clearly does—that there ought to be a number of works attributing the lack of national health insurance in the United States to the politics of race. As her own citations reveal, however, there are none. Similarly, very few accounts of the development of health care policy in Canada pay adequate attention to the role of territorial politics. Even fewer comparative works examining the two countries refer to either of these important factors in explaining the distinct trajectories of development of their health care systems. None points to these differences as providing an essential explanation for why the contemporary health care systems in the two countries look so different.

At the same time, health care remains a central issue in both countries. In 2005 poll respondents in both the United States and Canada ranked health care as the single most important domestic policy issue (Ipsos-Reid 2005, 18–19). Health care was a central fixture in the 2006 Canadian federal election. Health care reform was an important element of President Bush's 2006 State of the Union address and is already emerging in the 2008 Democratic presidential primaries. Health care has been at the top of the public policy agenda in both the United States and Canada now for more than a decade and a half. In both countries this current concern represents only a small segment of health care's distinguished pedigree as a long-standing public policy issue. Nearly a full century after national public health insurance was first proposed in the United States by Theodore Roosevelt in 1912 (and a half-decade later in Canada by the Liberal Party under William Lyon Mackenzie King), proposals for health care reform still abound. Understanding health care's long history is a crucial element in gaining perspective on current reforms. Beginning from very similar starting points prior to World War II, the provision of health care took divergent paths in the two countries in the middle of the twentieth century, with national public health insurance for hospital and physician services emerging in Canada while, in the United States, a system of public health insurance for seniors and those with low incomes developed alongside a system of private, primarily employer-provided health insurance. Comparing the two patterns of divergent development in these two countries with an otherwise relatively limited set of social, economic, and political differences deeply enriches our understanding of the historical development of health care in each country.

Health care is not simply a technical policy issue in either the United States or Canada; rather, public health insurance has been central to perceptions of national identity for both the United States and Canada. For many observers, both inside and outside the United States, the latter's status as the only western industrialized democracy without a system of universal public health insurance is often a central element in claims of American exceptionalism. The Canadian system of public health insurance is even more clearly an explicit element of national identity, which is especially crucial to claims of distinctiveness vis-à-vis the United States. Thus, an examination of the historical development of public health insurance in the two countries goes well beyond the issues generally perceived to be the province of public policy analysis. Such an examination implicates questions regarding who Americans and Canadians are as peoples, the magnitude and nature of the differences between them, and the underlying sources of those differences.

This work is intended to develop the argument that the politics of race in the United States and the politics of territorial integration in Canada together provide a powerful explanation of the divergent historical development of public health insurance in the two countries. This alternative interpretation is intended as a second opinion offered in contrast to more conventional wisdoms in each country. There is a widespread perception that health care systems in the United States and Canada present a stark contrast to each other. Differences in public health care, however, in the United States and Canada as well as the roots of these differences are more subtle and complex than generally recognized in academic policy analysis and popular debates. These differences, often exaggerated, caricaturized, and simplified, are widely believed to be rooted in fundamental differences in national values or political culture. The American system of targeted public health care and greater reliance on private provision of health care is often seen as evidence of the stronger influence in America of individualism and belief in a limited role for the state. Canada's universal public health care system is often taken as evidence of a greater Canadian predisposition toward collective provision of social well-being and acceptance of a greater role for the state. Alternatively, these differences are some-times seen as the result of the institutional distinctiveness of the political systems of the two countries—the fragmentation of power inherent in the American "separa-tion of powers" system vs. the relative concentration of power in the Canadian parliamentary system. These institutional differences are in turn usually explained as being rooted in divergent perceptions about the appropriate role of the state in each country. Finally, differences in public health insurance in the United States and Canada are sometimes explained as the result of path-dependent processes—hinging on earlier differences in the sequence and timing of the development of public health insurance, especially the development of private health benefits.

The central conclusion of this study is that the emergence of different systems of public health insurance in the United States and Canada was not predetermined by political culture, institutional configuration, or path dependence. Historical differ-ences between the two countries in public health care provision, which are at once both profound and subtle, are not easily explicable simply by reference to broad national-level cultural or institutional differences. Each was important; however, the key development of public health insurance in each country took place in a radically different social and political context—heavily shaped in one case by the politics of race and, in the other, by the politics of territory and language. The countries' divergent outcomes were strongly shaped by the intersection of public health insurance issues with other broad-scale social processes occurring at the same time—most notably, the extension of civil rights in the United States and the proc-ess of territorial integration in Canada.

In developing this argument, this work does not claim to present a definitive history of public health insurance in either country. It is, rather, an interpretation of that history. As such, the historical rendering here is far from comprehensive, and selected events and developments are emphasized to highlight particular pat-terns and illustrate specific themes—patterns and themes that contribute to argu-ments that, I hope, readers will find both provocative and compelling.

ACKNOWLEDGMENTS

I WOULD LIKE TO THANK all the people who provided helpful comments on the manuscript or various parts of it including Keith Banting, Colleen Grogan, Antonia Maioni, and Ted Marmor. My colleagues at the University of Waterloo and Wilfrid Laurier University—Sandra Burt, Colin Farrelly, and Debora VanNijnatten—were kind enough to read the manuscript in its early, unvarnished versions. Julie Simmons, Mark Sproule-Jones, and Debora VanNijnatten each afforded me the opportunity to lead graduate seminars on the manuscript material, which was invaluable in helping me organize and sharpen my arguments. Kevin Wipf, Andrew Banfield, Brad Ullner, and Matt Walcoff provided invaluable research assistance.

My thanks go to Tom Kent, former principal secretary to Prime Minister Lester B. Pearson, who kindly agreed to a personal interview that, as evident in the text, was extremely helpful. Monte Poen also kindly engaged in a long e-mail exchange that helped clarify a number of questions I had regarding the development of national health insurance proposals in the United States during the Truman era.

Parts of the manuscript were written while I held the Fulbright–Michigan State University Chair in Canadian Studies. For this, I would like to thank the Canada–U.S. Fulbright Program and its executive director, Michael Hawes. For welcoming me to MSU, I would like to thank Phil Handrick, Mike Unsworth, Alane Enyart, David Katz, and Catherine Yansa. In 2005 Duke University kindly hosted me as a visiting research professor at the Center for Canadian Studies. For their kindness during my stay, I thank Janice Engelhardt, Gilbert Merks, and John Herd Thompson.

I also am grateful to everyone at Georgetown University Press. Barry Rabe encouraged me to write this book and agreed to remain as editor emeritus through its final stages; I greatly appreciate this commitment. As many contributors to this series are well aware, Barry represents the gold standard for series editors. Gail Grella at Georgetown University Press was extremely patient and helpful in moving this manuscript along. Her consummate professionalism is greatly appreciated. Gail is simply the best acquisitions editor one could hope to have. My appreciation goes to two anonymous referees for their helpful and incisive comments that certainly contributed to strengthening the manuscript. I would especially like to thank James Morone for his invaluable comments, which were thoughtful, enthusiastic, and constructive. Although we have never met in person, in some important senses, he rescued the soul of the manuscript.

Finally, I would like to thank Debora VanNijnatten for her loving support of this and all my endeavors.

Of course, as always, any errors in fact or interpretation remain mine.

ABBREVIATIONS AND ACRONYMS

ADC	Aid to Dependent Children
AFDC	Aid to Families with Dependent Children
AHA	American Hospital Association
AMA	American Medical Association
BCMA	British Columbia Medical Association
BNA Act	British North America Act, 1867
BQ	Bloc Québécois
CCF	Cooperative Commonwealth Federation
CES	Committee on Economic Security
CHA	Canada Health Act, 1984
CHIA	Canadian Health Insurance Association
CHST	Canada Health and Social Transfer
CHT	Canada Health Transfer
CIHI	Canada Institutes for Health Information
CLIA	Canadian Life Insurance Association
CMA	Canadian Medical Association
CMAJ	Canadian Medical Association Journal
CPP	Canada Pension Plan
DHEW	Department of Health, Education, and Welfare
EPF	Established Programs Financing
ERISA	Employee Retirement Income Security Act
FLQ	Front de Libération du Québec
FSA	Federal Security Administration
HIPAA	Health Insurance Portability and Accountability Act
HMO	health maintenance organizations
IPA	individual practice association
JAMA	Journal of the American Medical Association
JNMA	Journal of the National Medical Association
MP	member of Parliament
NAACP	National Association for the Advancement of Colored People
NDP	New Democratic Party
NMA	National Medical Association
NPC	National Physicians Committee
OMA	Ontario Medical Association
PCCR	President's Committee on Civil Rights
POS	point-of-service plans
PPO	preferred provider organization
PQ	Parti Québécois

QPP   Québec Pension Plan
SCHIP   State Children's Health Insurance Program
SSA   Social Security Administration
UFA   United Farmers of Alberta

PART I

Introduction and Context

CHAPTER ONE

Explaining Public Health Insurance in the United States and Canada

Our goal is to ensure that Americans can choose and afford private health care coverage that best fits their individual needs. A government-run health care system is the wrong prescription. By keeping costs under control, expanding access, and helping more Americans afford coverage, we will preserve the system of private medicine that makes America's health care the best in the world.

President George W. Bush

We want a Canada where our universal health care system is a proud example of our national values at work. . . . Health care is the nation's first priority. Quality care; timely care. Care that is accessible regardless of income; portable right across Canada; and publicly funded. We are committed irrevocably to the principles of the Canada Health Act. They are part of who we are—a moral statement about fundamental fairness—that all Canadians should stand equal before our health care system."

Prime Minister Paul Martin

IN THE SECOND DEBATE of the 2004 presidential election, George W. Bush's strategy was to paint his opponent, John Kerry, as being out of step with American public opinion—characterizing Kerry as being on the "far left bank" of the American mainstream. In doing so, one of Bush's key targets was Kerry's proposed health care plan: "He said he's going to have a novel health care plan. You know what that is? The federal government is going to run it. It's the largest increase in federal government health care ever. And it fits with his philosophy. . . . That's what liberals do. They create government-sponsored health care. Maybe you think that makes sense. I don't." The charge prompted a forceful denial from Kerry in the third presidential debate: "It's not a government plan. The government doesn't require you to do anything." Beneath the rhetorical differences, the consensus between the two candidates against "government-run" health care was striking and emphasizes American exceptionalism—that is, the United States as the only industrialized country without universal health coverage.

3

A similar level of consensus was evident in the Canadian federal election of 2006; however, in this case, the consensus was in favor of protecting the Canadian system of universal public hospital and medical care insurance. All the major national parties agreed that public funding for health care had to be enriched, and all agreed that the basic principles of the existing system ought to be protected. Discussion of private-sector delivery of publicly funded health services—much less the private financing of health care—was verboten.

The distinctive tone of these debates and the starkly divergent consensus underpinning each highlight the differences in the politics of public health insurance between the two countries. What can these differences tell us about the exceptional development of public health insurance in the United States? What explains the existence of distinct health care systems in these two countries that, from a broader comparative perspective, seem so similar in so many other ways?

The Politics of Race in the United States

Sixty years ago, Swedish economist Gunnar Myrdal identified the problem of race as the central challenge facing American democracy—the essence of the "American dilemma." The reference to racial politics as an explanatory factor in public policy is not to imply that races exist in some objective sense. As Richard Iton notes, "While empirically races do not 'really' exist, the obsession with the implications of racial differences has affected the political activities of all Americans, in some manner, regardless of their background. As these categories have been imbued with significance, the behavior and perceptions of Americans have been affected so as to give even greater life to an essentially artificial realm" (2000, 20).

Concluding her own examination of the historical development of welfare policy in the United States a half century later, Jill Quadagno concluded that, in contrast to alternative interpretations of the central dynamic driving American society, "only Gunnar Myrdal has correctly identified the more important motor of change, the governing force from the nation's founding to the present: the politics of racial inequality" (1994, 188). More evocatively, Iton argues that "while it is tempting to view the existence of blacks in the United States as a minor issue at most, race is the ghost with a permanent seat at the table of American life, the spirit whose existence gives definition to all others" (2000, 236).

While the focus on race in American political science has waxed and waned and there continues to be significant debate about "just how much race matters in American politics," there is little doubt that it plays an important role (Hutchings and Valentino 2004, 383–84). Race has been an important factor in studies of partisanship and voting behavior, public opinion, the nature of representation, and the mass media (for an overview, see Hutchings and Valentino 2004). Race has also played an important role as an explanatory factor in public policy—especially in the area of welfare (see, for example, Brown 1999; Gilens 1999; Lieberman 1998; Mink 1995, 1998; Quadagno 1988, 1994; Williams 2003). Nevertheless, it remains true that "few analysts have argued that American exceptionalism—[including among other things] the lack of . . . a range of public goods and policies . . .

whether celebrated or cursed, is, to some significant degree, a function of American demographic heterogeneity, or simply race" (Iton 2000, 22; see also Quadagno 1994, 188).

No mainstream account of the historical development of public health insurance in the United States relies primarily on race in explaining why the health care system in the United States has taken the form it has. This oversight has been mirrored in the cross-national comparative literature on health care, with most examinations of the differences in the public provision of health care in Canada and the United States making little or no reference to race (see Vaillancourt-Rosenau 1992; Boase 1996; Hacker 1998, 2002; Maioni 1998; Tuohy 1999). At the same time, race has been an important factor in the analysis of the effects of the American health system and racially based health care disparities have been widely documented.[1]

There are two levels at which dynamics generated by the politics of race may help explain divergence in public health insurance policies in the United States and Canada. First, causal factors often used to explain divergent trajectories in health care policy in the United States and Canada may be explained, in turn, by the impact of the politics of race. For example, racial politics have been argued to have played a determining role in undermining the development of a conventional left in the American political system. More broadly, the individualist political culture in the United States has been argued to be, at root, a reflection of the politics of race (Quadagno 1994, 191–96; Iton 2000, 181).

While the indirect effects of racial politics on factors typically used to explain the development of public health insurance are important, the argument proposed here examines more-direct links between the politics of race and U.S. public policy. Among the most notable arguments in this genre is that the main barrier to public policy development in the United States can be traced to the role of race in southern politics and the resulting resistance to any federal programs that might challenge the racial status quo (Iton 2000, 150, 237). Using old-age pensions as an example of this dynamic in operation, Quadagno powerfully argues that "race was a key component in battles over New Deal policymaking" (1994, 10).[2] Given the institutional structure of the American federal system, this influence was transmitted to the national level through southern congressional representatives and as a result of the peculiarities of congressional operation—especially the control of key congressional committees—the magnitude of this influence was amplified.

Tracing the role of racial politics in public policy faces a significant challenge because many debates that implicate race are deeply coded. One of the most infamous examples is President Reagan's use of the term "welfare queens," which was widely understood as a reference to African American single mothers. As Quadagno argues, "Politicians say they are talking about social programs, but people understand that they're really taking about race. There is good reason for Americans to understand coded messages about social policy as substitutes for discussions of race, for real linkages between race and social policy exist" (1994, v). The challenge is to remain sensitive to the existence of racially coded terms and debates without succumbing to the temptation to read race into all debates.

The chapters in part II examine the degree to which such direct linkages between issues of race and the politics of health policy are evident in the history of public health insurance in the United States. The conclusion that these chapters draw is that race, through its interaction with other important causal factors, was a key element shaping the development of public health insurance in the United States. The politics of race were not a significant barrier to the development of public health insurance in the period from Theodore Roosevelt's commitment to national public health insurance in 1912 through the end of World War II. Had public health insurance been implemented in this period, almost certainly it would not have challenged the racial status quo. Southern Democrats in Congress retained powerful mechanisms to ensure that any new programs would not challenge segregation—the ability to make programs less racially inclusive where they were national (as in the case of Social Security), the option of leaving administration to state or local officials where programs were racially inclusive (as in the case of Aid to Families with Dependent Children), and the ability to block any nondiscrimination provisions. Had national public health insurance been implemented before World War II ended, it undoubtedly would have taken on a complexion similar to the other programs implemented in this period "when affirmative action was white"—that is, when major social programs were designed to confer advantage on whites (Katznelson 2005; Williams 2003).

Following a shift in the postwar period by which federal programs increasingly came to be linked with desegregation, the politics of race helped ensure that universal public health care was not adopted in the United States when such a system was emerging in Canada. In the immediate postwar period, the South's ability to enforce a policy of racial segregation on the federal government was being challenged, as was the racial status quo in the South. Because of the highly segregated nature of health services provision in the United States, it was virtually inevitable that the politics of public health insurance would become entwined with the politics of civil rights. This proved to be the case with President Harry S. Truman's attempts at national public health insurance, which demonstrated both that any new federal programs, including those for public health insurance, would be seen as a challenge to segregation in the South and that the southern coalition in concert with other oppositional forces still retained the political resources to resist such initiatives.

By the 1960s circumstances had changed dramatically as segregation in health care services went on the defensive even in the absence of federal health insurance programs. As a result, southern opposition to federal health insurance programs collapsed, paving the way for increased federal intervention with the emergence of Medicare and Medicaid in 1965. However, federal policymakers were not drawing on a clean slate. The reforms of the 1960s had been shaped in the late 1940s and early 1950s as federal policymakers struggled to find an approach to public health insurance that would allow them to overcome strong opposition from various quarters including the South—namely limiting the provision of public health insurance to the aged. Moreover, the politics of race even contributed to shaping specific design characteristics of the program as policymakers struggled with various options to ensure that southern doctors and hospitals would not boycott the new program—a possibility that would undoubtedly have placed its entire future in question. These concerns help explain the terms of the new programs, which were very favorable to physician and hospital interests but created serious cost-control problems that later would contribute to undermining the political viability of program expansion.

Issues relating to desegregation also contributed to decisions regarding how particular services were to be covered—most notably, adding a program of public health insurance for the needy and placing long-term nursing home care in the Medicaid program for the needy rather than the Medicare program for aged. The latter would have long-term implications for reinforcing the political viability of the Medicaid program—transferring it unintentionally from a program only for the needy disproportionately benefiting racial minorities to a middle-class program including large numbers of white seniors.

When debate turned to health insurance reform in the 1990s, the politics of race still lurked beneath the surface. The Clinton reformers carefully avoided igniting the issue of race in the health care discussions, and the initial Clinton reforms were carefully sold as benefiting the middle class and protecting middle-class health insurance coverage, rather than expanding coverage to those who did not have it. At the same time, racially charged debates about welfare and crime were heating up—fueled in part by the Clinton administration itself. Health reform itself was relatively insulated from the direct effects of racialized political dynamics, but these debates contributed to a context in which major national health insurance reforms were much less politically viable. Paradoxically, the intersection of the health care debates with the more highly racialized debates regarding welfare and crime control helps explain both why health insurance reform proceeded as far as it did and why it failed.

Territorial Politics in the Canadian Federation

As race has been the ghost with a permanent seat at the table of American political life, territorial integration has always been and continues to be the central issue of Canadian statecraft. As a result of the interplay of powerful territorially defined dynamics resulting from cultural, linguistic, and economic tensions in the Canadian federation, "Canada is a rich case study in the subtle interplay between territorial politics and the welfare state. The combination of federal institutions, linguistic and cultural pluralism, and regional conflicts has important implications for the design of Canadian social programs" (Banting 1995, 271). While territorial politics cannot be reduced to tensions between the English-speaking majority in Canada and the French-speaking minority primarily in Québec, the politics of this ethnolinguistic divide has been the most powerful of these Canadian political cleavages.

As testament to the immediacy of territorial politics in Canada, a referendum on the issue of Québec sovereignty was held in Québec in 1995—an earlier one having been held in 1980—and was defeated by only the narrowest of margins: 50.6 percent to 49.4 percent.[3] Underpinning these more recent manifestations, territorial politics have deep roots in the history of the Canadian federation. Dynamics generated by the politics of territorial integration significantly shaped policy debates in the postwar period, and coincident with the hospital and medical care insurance debates, their full weight came to bear on Canadian politics in the late 1950s and early 1960s.

Despite obvious and crucial differences, these ethnolinguistic cleavages in Canada share important characteristics with the racial divide in the United States. Both relate primarily to the politics of identity in which the characteristics of and inclusion in both majority and minority groups is socially constructed. Both also related historically to an essentialist politics of inclusion and exclusion that buttressed a system of unequal power relations between majority and minority groups. At the same time, a notable difference between the politics of race in the United States and the politics of language in Canada lies in the degree to which these societal cleavages in Canada have aligned with territorial boundaries. Subnational territorial boundaries in Canada coincide with major cultural and linguistic divisions—most notably in the case of Québec. More than 80 percent of the population of the province of Québec is comprised of mother-tongue French speakers. At the same time, more than 85 percent of Canada's French-speaking population lives in Québec (Boychuk 2008). Québec constitutes a distinct, predominantly French-speaking society within Canada.

This alignment of territorial boundaries and cultural and linguistic cleavages allowed Canada's French-speaking minority to maintain control of a crucial lever of institutional power. Concern over linguistic and cultural assimilation within English-speaking North America has resulted in strong popular and elite attachment in Québec to the provincial government—as opposed to the federal government—as a bulwark against assimilationist pressures. As illustrated above, Québec nationalism as it operates in this institutional context continues to pose a significant challenge to the existence of the Canadian federal state.

Canada is also marked by sharp economic tensions among various regions, which also reinforce territorial divisions. Two types of interregional economic tensions exist. First, there are inherent tensions between provinces whose economies rely primarily on an industrial base (especially Ontario and Québec) and provinces whose economies rely primarily on natural resource extraction such as petroleum (Alberta), agriculture (Saskatchewan), and fishing and forestry (Atlantic Canada). Second, inherent tensions lie in the relationship between richer provinces and poorer provinces, especially in regard to the interregional redistribution of wealth by the federal government.[4]

These territorially based axes of political conflict have been reinforced by existing institutions—especially Canadian federalism. Federal institutions not only reflect but also reinforce and invigorate these territorial axes of political cleavage as these institutions are particularly responsive to political claims that can be cast in territorial terms (Porter 1965). Although both cultural/linguistic and economic tensions have histories that predate Canadian confederation, these tensions remain powerfully in operation.

In this context, social policies have long been recognized as important mechanisms of social integration. In societies where the primary social cleavages were along class lines, social policies were central to mediating class divisions (Banting 1995, 270). Similarly, in societies marked by territorially based axes of political conflict, social policies also play a central role in the politics of territorial integration. Social programs are crucial in creating direct connections between citizens and their governments, helping provide legitimacy for those governments, as well as helping to foster a sense of community by defining the relevant sharing community on which claims can be made and to whose members a debt of obligation is owed (Titmuss 1970). Thus, it is not surprising that social policy in Canada has been swept up in the political struggles generated by territorial challenges to the integrity of the federal state. In the postwar period, federal policymakers recognized national social programs as potentially potent tools to defend against these territorial challenges—a point of which provincial officials were also highly cognizant.

In the context of welfare state expansion, a dynamic of competitive state-building, in which the different orders of government compete vigorously to occupy political and policy space, would come to dominate. Banting explains why:

> Social programs controlled by the central government can become instruments of nation building, helping to mediate regional tensions and strengthen the state against centrifugal forces rooted in territorial politics. Alternatively, social programs designed and controlled at the regional level can become instruments for strengthening regional cultures and enhancing the significance of local communities in the lives of citizens, thereby reinforcing differentiation and centrifugal tendencies at the national level. (1995, 270)

The link between social programs and the politics of territory would be most evident in the clashes between the provincial government of Québec and the federal government from the mid-1940s through the maturation of the welfare state in the 1970s. The intensity of these battles "can be understood only by appreciating the extent to which the two governments vied to retain the loyalty of Quebecers and to protect and enhance their institutional power" (Banting 1995, 284). At the same time, the reliance of poorer provinces on interregional redistribution by the federal government, including through national social programs, has generated a potent contradictory dynamic and powerful institutional support for an expansive role for the federal government through national social policy.

Public health insurance in Canada has been strongly shaped by the politics of territorial integration, including the imperative of the federal government to ensure the territorial integrity of the Canadian polity—especially in response to the challenges posed by secessionist tendencies in Québec. On the one hand, federal intervention in health care offered the opportunity for the federal government to create a direct connection with individual citizens in the disparate regions of Canada and foster a sense of attachment between them and the national polity. On the other hand, recognition of the potential role of social policy in nation-building prompted strenuous resistance on the part of certain provinces—most notably Québec—to new federal health insurance programs.

Despite provincial efforts at reform in the post–World War I era, marked most notably by the recommendations of a Royal Commission in British Columbia in 1919 in favor of compulsory public health insurance, commitments by the federal Liberal Party in 1919 to compulsory national health insurance, and further provincial experimentation with compulsory health insurance in the context of the Great Depression, serious efforts at reform would not emerge until World War II. In the immediate postwar period, an emergent vision for a national program of public, comprehensive, universal health insurance and even a more limited plan foundered in the face of resistance from Québec as the federal and provincial government struggled over control of this tool of state-building. Provincial plans for public hospital insurance such as the one that developed in Saskatchewan emerged out of this collapse largely as a matter of historical accident. Following the advent of these earlier provincial plans, a national hospital insurance plan emerged only as the result of a cycle of political one-upmanship between the federal government and Ontario in the latter half of the 1950s rather than by some overall design or inexorable logic.

In the 1960s, in the face of growing nationalist sentiment in Québec and a coherent overall strategy on the part of the Québec government to become *maître chez nous* ("master in our own house"), physician care insurance emerged as a federal initiative to rebalance a series of decisions that had tilted social policy dominance strongly toward the provincial government (Boychuk and Banting 2008). Implemented in the face of resistance from the Québec government that, in contrast to 1945, would be unsuccessful, the addition of a national program for cost-sharing physician care insurance to the program of hospital care insurance laid the basis for the Canadian public health insurance system as it exists today.

The public system began to erode, however, in the English-speaking provinces, especially in the late 1970s. This became a serious political liability for the federal government in the context of the Québec referendum on sovereignty-association in 1980 in which the federal government aimed to portray itself as the guarantor of social rights and social programs in Canada. (Sovereignty-association was a proposal to combine political sovereignty for Québec with continued economic association with the rest of Canada.) In the wake of the 1980 Québec referendum, the federal government reasserted its role in hospital and physician care insurance through the Canada Health Act of 1984 (CHA).

Against the backdrop of Canadian debates regarding deepening economic integration with the United States (Canada–U.S. Free Trade in 1987–88 and the North American Free Trade Agreement in 1993), in which the sustainability of public health insurance would figure prominently, the Canadian health care system—symbolized by the Canada Health Act—came to enjoy iconic status, especially in English Canada.

In the wake of the Québec 1995 referendum, the federal government began another attempt to reinvigorate its role in health care as it had in the wake of the first Québec referendum—positioning itself as the guarantor of social rights in Canada, the defender of the CHA, and proposing initiatives to consolidate and extend the scope of the public health insurance model. These initiatives included proposals to extend coverage for prescription drugs and home care and, later, to provide national wait-time guarantees for services provided under the public system. None of these efforts was successful, and the federal struggle to reassert its role in this field continues. Throughout, the politics of territorial integration have remained central.

Existing Explanations

The central explanations for differences in public health insurance in the United States and Canada, in the literature on this subject, pay little or no attention to the politics of race or the politics of territorial integration. Conventional explanations often attribute differences between the two countries to the distinct political cultures or political institutions of the two countries. More recent explanations draw on historical institutionalism and, especially, the concept of path dependence.

Political Culture

Political cultural arguments are epitomized by Lipset's well-known formulation: "The two countries differ in their basic organizing principles. Canada has been and is a more class-aware, elitist, law-abiding, statist, collectivity-oriented, and particularistic (group-oriented) society than the United States" (1990, 8). Lipset argues that "the differences between the two countries are particularly striking with respect to the role of government in medical care" (1990, 138).[5] Following this type of argument, Kudrle and Marmor (1981, 111) give explanatory preeminence to ideological differences between the two countries:

> In every policy area it appears that general public as well as elite opinion was at least as supportive of state action in Canada as in the United States at a given time and often, as in the case of public health-care, considerably more supportive. This support appears to underlie not just the typically earlier enactment of policy in Canada but also subsequent changes [including] the rapid development of Medicare after hospital insurance.

Thus, their overall conclusion is that "the ideological difference—slight by international standards—between Canada and the United States appears to have made a considerable difference in welfare state development" (Kudrle and Marmor 1981, 112).

Interest group politics are also argued to have been conditioned by the political culture of each country.[6] For example, Tuohy argues that physicians' perceptions of their own interests—especially as represented by the Canadian Medical Association (CMA) and the American Medical Association (AMA)—were substantially different in the two countries and that such differences reflected broader differences in political culture: "One of the key manifestations of the 'tory streak' in the health care arena in Canada . . . has been in patterns of *medical* opinion, and in positions taken by organized medicine at critical junctures and in the ongoing playing out of the logic of the respective systems" (1999, 117). In this interpretation, the cultural pre-disposition of the Canadian medical profession explains why it was supportive of universal public health insurance in the 1940s while the AMA was not.

Political Institutions

Formal political institutions have also long been argued to be key to explaining divergence in public health insurance in the two countries. The most common explanation for the slow and limited development of public health insurance cover-age in the United States is the role of interest groups—especially the AMA—operating in a context of high levels of institutional fragmentation (Marmor 1973; Morone 1990, 255–56; Quadagno 2005; Starr 1982, 279, 369). These explanations typically focus on the American presidential system and weak political parties—the corollary of the separation of legislative and executive powers. According to this perspective, the failures of past efforts at health care reform in the United States were largely predetermined, and differences between the two countries are most clearly the result of continuing distinctiveness of institutional configuration: "It is unlikely that the U.S. will ever adopt national health insurance at the federal level because of differences in their respective political systems" (Vaillancourt-Rosenau 1992, 2). One of the strongest statements of this position is Steinmo and Watts's provocative title, "It's the Institutions, Stupid!" (Steinmo and Watts 1995).

Certainly, the U.S. and Canadian public health insurance systems are embedded in the larger institutional structures of each country, which exhibit important simi-larities and differences. The two broadest institutional differences are the relation-ship between the executive and the legislature branches in the two countries and the system of federalism in each. In the United States, the separation of powers system constitutionally prohibits the president from being a member of the legisla-ture. While the president may initiate legislation indirectly through congressional members, Congress is responsible for passing legislation.[7] The president, as the head of the executive branch, administers and applies legislation.

In Canada, in contrast, the powers of the executive and legislature are fused. The prime minister and his appointed cabinet of ministers are elected members of the legislature and must command the support of a majority of seats in the Parliament. Under majority governments (where one party directly controls a majority of par-liamentary seats), the government (prime minister and cabinet) generally has the ability to pass any legislation it wishes as a result of strong party discipline—a situation in which the prime minister and cabinet retain relatively strict control over individual members of Parliament (MPs) belonging to their party. Cabinet ministers are expected to publicly support collective cabinet decisions (cabinet soli-darity) and are not permitted to publicly disclose positions they or their colleagues have taken in cabinet discussions (cabinet secrecy). While this system serves to concentrate the electoral accountability of the governing party (the leadership of the governing party is solely responsible for all legislation passed under its tenure), it creates a policymaking process that is considerably less transparent than in the United States. In Canada much of the political bargaining over legislation that takes place openly in the United States—between the president and Congress, between the two houses of Congress, and between individual members of each house—takes place under the cloak of cabinet secrecy (Banting 1987, 82).

Furthermore, while both systems are federal, there are important differences between the two. In the United States, state interests are represented intergovernmentally by the state governments and intragovernmentally at the federal level in the U.S. Senate. Because of this arrangement, the federal government in the United States has been more able to legitimately claim the mantle of national government. The American federal system has developed since the adoption of the American Constitution in 1789 into a much more centralized federation. While hewing to the constitutional requirement of federalism that each order of government is constitutionally independent of the other and constitutionally equal to the other, there is little doubt in the United States that the federal government now enjoys a superordinate status relative to the states.

In contrast, the Canadian system has developed into a much more decentralized federal system than anticipated by the Canadian fathers of Confederation who saw the provinces as little more than aggrandized municipalities. Two important factors contributed to this pattern of development: inadequate mechanisms of intragovernmental representation of regional interests within the federal level of government and the existence of a territorially defined, linguistically distinct community with strong (though not unchallenged) claims to nationhood in the province of Québec. In regard to the former, the Canadian Senate was based on rough parity between regions in Canada (Atlantic Canada, Québec, Ontario, and the west). However, as the Senate was (and remains) unelected, it lacked political legitimacy to challenge the elected lower house in the Canadian bicameral system, the House of Commons. As a result, the Senate has largely become anachronistic and exercises little real power over legislation in Canada—despite the occasional exception proving the rule.

The corollary has been that regional interests have had to find expression elsewhere—namely, through provincial governments. A central dynamic reinforcing the power of the provinces has been the role played by Québec. On the assumption that its interests were best served by ensuring that decisions important to its cultural integrity were made at the provincial level (with French-speaking Québécois constituting a minority of the population in Canada but a majority of the population inside the province), Québec has consistently and powerfully defended provincial jurisdiction as set out in the British North America Act of 1867 (BNA Act). Furthermore, it has pushed for an expansion of provincial influence where possible. Joined in this endeavor to varying degrees by other provinces, Québec has attained considerable success in this strategy. The result has been that Canadian provinces are far more powerful vis-à-vis the federal government than the states are in the USA.

The different levels of centralization in the two countries' federal systems is evident in their respective systems of public health insurance. The Canadian health care system is highly decentralized. Provinces are granted the preponderance of jurisdictional authority for health care under the Canadian constitution.[8] Primary jurisdiction over health care was granted to the provinces by S. 92 of the British

North America Act (later to become the Constitution Act of 1982) that assigned the provinces jurisdiction over the "Establishment, Maintenance, and Management of Hospitals." The federal government has involved itself in the provision of health care, however, primarily through the use of the federal spending power. This power, which is not explicitly established in the Canadian constitution but has recently been recognized by the federal and provincial governments under the Social Union Framework Agreement of 1999, allows the federal government to make transfers to the provinces attaching whatever conditions it wishes so long as it does not undertake to legislate directly within a field of provincial jurisdiction. This power underpins the CHA, which is the legislative basis of the Canadian health care system.

Primary responsibility for publicly provided health care resides with the American states by virtue of the Tenth Amendment, which declares that any powers not constitutionally delegated to the federal government are reserved for the states. However, a central role for the federal government in health care provision has evolved through its taxing power (e.g., providing tax subsidies for employer-sponsored health insurance coverage), spending power (e.g., making conditional transfers to the states under programs such as Medicaid), and power to regulate interstate commerce (e.g., prohibiting states from regulating health insurance provided by self-insuring employers). Through these mechanisms, the federal government plays a more direct and immediate role in shaping public health insurance in the United States than has been the case for the federal government in Canada. Given these important institutional differences, it is not surprising that numerous accounts of the divergent development of public health insurance in the two countries make reference to them.

Historical Institutionalism

The most recent academic literature goes beyond a simple focus on the distinctiveness of formal political institutions and, in explaining the differences in public health insurance in the two countries, draws heavily on the historical institutionalist approach (Hacker 1998, 2002; Maioni 1998; Tuohy 1999). This approach focuses on the unfolding of the policy development over time, including the effects of policies and institutions in shaping the politics of a policy field. Historical institutionalist approaches are marked by two main characteristics. First, they "'take time seriously', specifying sequences and tracing transformations and processes of varying context and temporality" (Pierson and Skocpol 2002, 695). Second, historical institutionalists "analyze macro contexts and hypothesize about the combined effects of institutions and processes rather than examining just one institution or process at a time" (696). Historical institutionalism treats history as a process that evolves—emphasizing the operation of causal linkages over time (699).

Path dependence is increasingly a central concept in the historical institutional approach. In turn, critical junctures, sequencing, and positive feedback are crucial elements in the overall concept of path dependence.[9] The starting point in the unfolding of a path-dependent process is a critical juncture or choice point. At critical junctures, change becomes possible. Perhaps described most aptly by John

Kingdon, critical junctures occur when a confluence of events opens a "window of opportunity" for change to take place.[10] At these critical junctures, the options for policy change are, at least relatively, open and contingent. They are *critical* junctures precisely because constraints on policy are loosened and different pathways may be chosen.

Second, sequencing, the order in which events happen, is important in determining outcomes. A different sequence of the exact same events may result in a substantially different outcome (Pierson 2004, 18, 66, 68). A good illustration of this is the common path-dependence argument that events occurring earlier in the causal sequence will generally have greater impact than events occurring later (Thelen 2003, 219; Pierson 2004, 18)

An additional important concept related to timing and sequencing is conjuncture or intercurrence—how the timing of a critical juncture in one process fits with the timing and sequence of other distinct but simultaneously unfolding processes (Pierson 2004, 55).[11] A final central element of path dependence is positive feedback—earlier policy outcomes creating conditions favorable to further development along an existing path. At the same time, development along a given path may also constrain the range of possible paths of development. In the strongest versions of path dependence, this creates "lock-in."

Combined, these separate elements generate a unified conception of policy development—path dependence. In this conception, "politics . . . involves some elements of chance (agency, choice) but . . . once a path is taken, once-viable alternatives become increasingly remote, as all the relevant actors adjust their strategies to accommodate the prevailing pattern." The combination of "some contingency at the front end and some degree of determinism at the back end of path-dependent processes" results in patterns of historical development that may be characterized as "punctuated equilibrium"—"moments of 'openness' and rapid innovation followed by long periods of institutional stasis or 'lock in'" (Thelen 2003, 219, 209).[12] In contrast to the imagery of punctuated equilibrium, more recent models of evolutionary change have focused on policy drift, policy conversion, layering, and subterranean policy changes (see Thelen 2003; Hacker 2004; Boychuk and Banting 2008).

Recent examinations of divergence in the U.S. and Canadian health care systems, which draw heavily on historical institutionalism and path dependence, have a number of common threads (Hacker 1998, 2002; Maioni 1998; Tuohy 1999). First, public health insurance in the two countries is typically seen as having developed from a roughly common starting point. At that time, it seemed plausible that they might follow the same path of development. Then different developments took place in each country that launched each on a distinctive path. These differences then became self-reinforcing so that, over time, the two countries increasingly diverged.

In order to provide powerful explanations of differences across countries, a historical institutional interpretation must establish that at least one of the two countries could have adopted the path taken by the other if it were not for some contingent event. An emphasis on the broad similarities between the two countries is not important merely in establishing a most-similar-case methodology; it is also necessary for implying contingency at critical junctures. Tuohy's account of the development of distinct systems of health insurance in Canada and the United States is a good example of a historical institutional interpretation that places heavy explanatory weight on contingency. For Tuohy the emergence of different systems of health insurance ultimately comes down to the accident of strategic miscalculation by proponents of reform in the United States. First, American states did not become the "loci of experimentation with governmental hospital insurance" as was the case in the Canadian provinces because of policy inertia in the American states, which led reformers to focus their efforts at the national level. This strategic choice, if made differently, could have led to similar outcomes in the two countries, according to Tuohy (1999, 47–48).

Another key factor for Tuohy is that Democratic policymakers failed to push for universal national health insurance in 1965 in the wake of the Johnson landslide:

> What needs to be explained in the US case . . . is why a comprehensive universal plan was not adopted *in the 1960s*—particularly when, under similar conditions in the health care arena, such a plan was adopted in Canada. . . . All else flows from this critical moment. If the United States had a health care arena like no other in the 1990s, that was the result of the logic of the system left in place by the decision not to adopt comprehensive universal health insurance in the 1960s. (1999, 118)

In Tuohy's judgment, "it is quite conceivable that had a different strategic judgment been made and the introduction of universal national health insurance had been attempted, the subsequent history of American health policy would have been very different" (1999, 120).

Second, the timing of events in the development of public health insurance is critical in historical institutionalist accounts in terms of both sequencing (the order in which events occurred) as well as conjunctures (the intercurrence of developments in public health insurance with other processes occurring in the broader political realm). Hacker develops an impressive version of the importance of sequencing in public health insurance reform:

> Three questions of sequence are particularly important in determining the path countries eventually take: whether governments fail to enact national health insurance before a sizable proportion of the public enrolled in physician-dominated private insurance plans, whether initial public insurance programs are focused on residual populations such as the elderly and the very poor, and whether efforts to build up the medical industry preceded the universalization of access. Countries that do all these things, as the United States did, are left facing virtually insuperable political barriers to the passage of national health insurance. (1998, 128)

Once a significant majority of Americans were covered by voluntary private health insurance arrangements (primarily on an employment-related basis), the extension of compulsory public health insurance to this portion of the population faced steep political barriers. Similarly, once efforts to build up the medical industry had been successfully undertaken, efforts to significantly reorganize relations in the sector faced much more serious obstacles. Finally, public insurance offered to particular categories of people is argued to have removed the most pressing arguments for universal insurance—the need for coverage for the aged and those with low incomes—from the arsenal of reform proponents. Hacker argues that differences in the degree of private voluntary insurance coverage were key in shaping the distinct trajectories of public health insurance development in the United States and Canada (2002, 248).

In terms of conjunctures, the interaction between public health insurance development and broader political factors is strongly stressed in Tuohy's emphasis on the "accidental" nature of the systems: "Key features of health care systems are 'accidental' in the sense that they were shaped by ideas and agendas in place at the time a window of opportunity was opened by factors in the broader political system" (Tuohy 1999, 6). As a result, "the systems that resulted were largely, if not entirely, 'accidents' of the timing of their birth—had windows opened at different times, they might have looked quite different" (1999, 239). More specifically, she argues that

> Canadian medicare bears the marks of its birth in the 1960s, an era of high public expectations and government expansiveness, in which the indemnity model of private insurance had become established and the public underwriting of the costs of a professionally dominated system appeared feasible. The U.S. Medicare and Medicaid systems were born in the same period, and were fashioned on a similar model. But . . . they were introduced in a national context in which the legacy of past policy failures conditioned policy-makers to adopt an incremental approach that ironically sowed the seeds of future policy failures (1999, 32).[13]

Third, a central element of historical institutionalist interpretations is policy feedback—the recognition that health insurance policy itself contributed significantly to shaping the subsequent political struggles over policy (Hacker 1998, 82; Maioni 1998, esp. ch. 8; Tuohy 1999). Whereas such processes can be transformational, typically in the health policy literature they have been depicted as being self-reinforcing—contributing to path dependence and lock-in.

Categorical programs, Medicare and Medicaid, are argued to have stemmed the tide in the United States for more radical policy innovation such as universal health insurance—effects that have been argued to have been relatively automatic, if not inevitable (Hacker 1998, 128; Maioni 1998, 165). For Hacker, the focus of initial public programs on residual populations such as the aged or the poor had three effects that stemmed further development of universal public health insurance: initial programs were expensive because the cost of covering the elderly and poor are very high; they focused on groups largely outside the mainstream of the economy; and finally, both public health insurance for the aged and poor piggybacked on existing programs (Social Security and Aid to Families with Dependent Children [AFDC]) to which their political fortunes became closely tied (1998, 128). For Maioni, policy outcomes in the 1960s, which were strongly shaped by earlier developments, in turn "created very different settings for the politics of health care in subsequent decades by changing the incentives and interests of actors and groups in the policy process" (1998, 7). Following this emphasis on "lock-in," Tuohy's account also rests quite heavily on determinism after the initial critical juncture. She examines how policies "have their 'legatory' effect—not simply by habit or accustomation, but rather through the logics that they establish, logics with their own dynamics that over time can either reinforce or transform the structural and institutional characteristics of the health care system" (1999, 124).

A Better Vantage Point

Of these three broad variants of explanations of the differences of health insurance in the United States and Canada—political culture, political institutions, and historical institutionalism—none adequately considers the role of the politics of race in the former and the politics of territorial integration in the latter. As argued below, examining health insurance in the United States from the comparative vantage point provided by the divergent developments in Canada highlights the weaknesses of these conventional explanations for American exceptionalism. Moreover, the Canadian case provides an analogous example of how health policy development became inextricably entwined with other, broad-scale political processes unfolding at the same time.

Overview of the Book

Chapter 2 highlights the different contexts in the two countries at the outset of the period in which attempts at public health insurance reforms initially took place. At the same time, the chapter outlines the similarities between early reform attempts in both. It provides a brief overview of the numerous failed efforts at health insurance reform at both the national level and state/provincial level in the United States and Canada from 1910 to 1940. The chapter highlights the degree to which the politics, rhetoric, and tenor of these debates in the two countries were very similar—emphasizing the similarities, rather than differences, in political cultures. Moreover, the outcomes were also similar—highlighting not the institutional differences in executive–legislature relations in the two countries but, rather, the similarities in how the states and provinces were constrained from acting in the face of federal inaction.

Parts II and III, which focus on the United States and Canada, respectively, outline the divergence between the health care systems of the two countries in the immediate postwar period through their maturation. Part II focuses on the role of the politics of race in shaping the development of public health insurance in the United States. Chapter 3 examines failed attempts at health care reform in the United States during the Truman era—focusing on how the intersection of the politics of health care and the politics of civil rights helped ensure the failure of these reforms. Chapter 4 examines the development of Medicare/Medicaid in the 1960s, arguing that important elements of the Medicare compromise resulted from the impact of racial politics and that these compromises set the stage for the failure of further reforms over the following decade. Chapter 5 examines the role of race in shaping the politics of the Clinton reforms in the 1990s, arguing that the particular intersection of race and health care politics—which was much different than in earlier periods—helps explain why health insurance reform proceeded as far as it did and why it failed.

Part III complements the analysis in part II by using divergent developments in Canada to highlight the weaknesses in conventional interpretations of American exceptionalism. Before World War II efforts at health insurance reform in the United States and Canada ended at much the same place, with reforms at both the federal and state/provincial levels having been defeated. As World War II drew to a close, attempts at reform were again undertaken at both levels in each country. In this period public health insurance in the United States and Canada became more tightly bound up with the politics of race and territorial integration in each country, respectively, and the difference in outcomes was striking. While initial postwar efforts at federal reform in Canada largely failed, as they had in the United States, successful reform was undertaken in the province of Saskatchewan (and later in British Columbia) while similar efforts again failed in the American states. A decade later a national system of universal hospital insurance finally came to fruition, followed by universal public medical care insurance yet a decade later. Chapters 6, 7, and 8 outline the development of this national system of public hospital and medical care insurance in Canada.

An examination of this outcome in Canada sheds a powerful light on the development of public health insurance in the United States. These distinct cross-national patterns of development highlight the weaknesses in conventional explanations of American health insurance exceptionalism, including those that focus on considerations of political culture, institutional design, and path dependence—none of which, on their own, provides adequate explanations for these divergent trajectories of development in public health insurance. In doing so, this comparison buttresses the argument, outlined in part II, that adequate understandings of the development of public health insurance in the United States must go beyond these factors to incorporate a consideration of the politics of race.

At the same time, the Canadian case provides a parallel illustration of the importance of dynamics related to the politics of identity in shaping the broader development of the welfare state. In Canada, the primary (though not only) axis of territorial conflict centered on an ethnolinguistic construction of group difference that generated strains on the federal state and, in turn, created a context in which the federal government would attempt to wield national social policy in the pursuit of territorial integration. While the racial divide in the United States and the ethnolinguistic divide in Canada each played out in highly distinctive ways in their respective national contexts, in neither case could these crucial axes of conflict in the politics of health insurance be reduced simply to class, ideology, or material self-interest. Rather, they were related to socially constructed politics of identity. Most important, in neither case were the politics of health insurance self-contained or insulated from these broader political dynamics.

The central argument of these chapters is that the development of national universal public hospital and medical care insurance in Canada was tightly linked with broader political processes unfolding at the same time—most notably, the politics of the ethnolinguistic divide and the attendant process of national territorial integration. The development of public health insurance was not a smooth evolution in which these programs emerged naturally from Canadian political culture, the parliamentary fusion-of-powers, distinctive Canadian federal arrangements, or path-dependent processes set in motion by the adoption of public hospital insurance in Saskatchewan in 1947. The process was tenuous and contingent, and at numerous points, the development of a system of health insurance much more closely approximating that of the United States was a strong possibility. The crucial element driving the Canadian health insurance system in a direction distinct from that taken by the United States was the conjuncture at key points between the politics of health care and the politics of territorial integration. The latter played a crucial role in contributing to the emergence of universal public insurance—just as the politics of race played a key role in forestalling universal public health insurance in the United States.

Chapter 6 examines the failure of federal reform in the immediate postwar period, which mirrored developments in the United States. In both cases, sectional interests used critical institutional levers of power to oppose the development of national programs of health insurance that threatened to intrude on established social relations in a particular region. However, because in Canada the constraining effects of federalism were briefly lifted on reform in the provinces, universal public hospital insurance was implemented in Saskatchewan and, later, British Columbia. Chapter 7 examines the development of a national program of public hospital insurance in Canada a decade later. The chapter argues that this development, while highly contingent, provides a contrasting perspective on path-dependent interpretations of what took place in the United States. The chapter also highlights the degree to which certain elements later seen as central to the Canadian public health insurance model—especially universality and first-dollar coverage—were incidental in the original version of public health insurance. Chapter 8 examines the extension of public health insurance coverage to physician care, emphasizing the degree to which the politics of public health insurance were tightly enmeshed with the politics of territorial integration—the latter generating a powerful dynamic auguring for an expanded federal role that ultimately led to universal public hospital and physician care insurance as it exists in Canada today. Chapter 9 examines the rise of public health insurance to iconic status in Canada as well as looking at the extent to which territorial politics remain central in the politics of health care reform.

In part IV I consider the implications of the alternative interpretation posited in these chapters. Chapter 10 outlines the similarities and differences in the contemporary American and Canadian systems of public health insurance. Although the differences between the two are clearly significant, the chapter argues that they are considerably more complex and nuanced than is often assumed—reflecting the complex path of development of each system and the degree to which public insurance in each country has been indelibly marked by the context of its development. Chapter 11 considers the theoretical and conceptual implications of this reinterpretation as well as its implications for policy development. The chapter argues that this reading of the history of health care reform in the United States suggests that, although complications related to the politics of race remain latent, the latitude for health care reform may be wider than often thought. It also argues that territorial politics remain central to the future of public health insurance in Canada and that this dynamic, which has underpinned the stasis in the current system, also could generate radical change. In both cases, the dynamics that help explain the historical development of public health insurance in the United States and Canada—the politics of race and the politics of territorial integration—will remain central to their future.

CHAPTER TWO

Similar Beginnings, Different Contexts, 1910–40

I expected to find a contest between a government and a people: I found two nations warring in the bosom of a single state: I found a struggle, not of principles, but of races. . . .

Lord Durham

Health insurance will constitute the next great step in social legislation.

Dr. Rupert Blue, U.S. Surgeon General

M ANY READERS may be surprised to find that it was an observer of Canadian politics who would in 1839 refer to a war between the "races"—a reference to linguistic and territorial tensions that would still be starkly evident in the Canadian federal system nearly eighty years later when public health insurance reform would first emerge on the political agenda. While public health insurance debates in Canada took place in the context of recurrent and sometimes incendiary tensions between English Canada and a French-speaking national community primarily centered in Québec, public health insurance proposals in the United States emerged on the heels of the development of racial segregation in the southern states that, unsurprisingly, extended to health services. Because of the different institutional and political contexts in which racial and linguistic tensions would play out, the intersection of these contexts and the politics of health care would take significantly different forms in the two countries. Nevertheless, in their respective national contexts, these dynamics would be crucial in shaping the development of public health insurance.

Many readers may also be surprised that the prediction of the imminent adoption of public health insurance at the end of the first decade of the twentieth century was made by an American—the U.S. surgeon general no less. Beginning in the early 1910s efforts at health insurance reform occurred at both the national and state/provincial level, first in the United States and somewhat later in Canada. Over the next thirty years the pattern of development in the two countries was remarkably similar, and reform efforts at the national and state/provincial levels followed roughly the same chronology. Moreover, the tenor of the health reform debates in the two countries was similar. Finally, the outcomes also were similar: efforts to implement public health insurance in this period failed at the federal and state/provincial levels in both the United States and Canada.

The American Context and Public Health Insurance Initiatives, 1910–45

At the time that the issue of national health insurance emerged on the political landscape in the United States in the early decades of the twentieth century, the system of racial segregation in the South had been only recently consolidated. Segregationist policies had been evident immediately following the Civil War including, for example, the Black Codes. However, in the Reconstruction period, the development of segregation was relatively limited, and rights were extended to African Americans under legislation such as the Civil Rights Act of 1875, which presaged similar legislation to be adopted nearly a century later. With the removal of Union troops in 1877, the South was left to its own devices in determining how race relations would be managed, and in 1883 the Supreme Court struck down in the 1875 Civil Rights Act. Following these changes, a system of pervasive and strictly enforced racial segregation embodied not only in social practices but encoded in state legislation developed. As a legal system, Jim Crow would receive constitutional legitimacy from the Supreme Court in 1896, which helped pave the way for the further entrenchment of this system of racial apartheid.

As this system developed, so simultaneously did a political configuration capable of defending this "southern way of life." This configuration included the adoption of particular patterns of political organization that functioned to maximize the influence of whites in the South and, simultaneously, the influence of the South in national politics. The first of these patterns was the disenfranchisement of African Americans. The second was the pattern of solid electoral support among white southerners for the Democratic Party.

These two patterns contributed to greatly leveraging the influence of southern Democrats in Congress. First, the rules of the Senate required a majority of two-thirds to override a filibuster. With seventeen southern states, the South thus had the ability to block federal legislation. Second, in both the House of Representatives and the Senate, committee membership and chairmanships were determined on the basis of seniority. In the absence of electoral competition outside of the all-white primaries, Democratic representatives in the South were typically of long tenure, allowing them to accede to senior posts in the committee system. This also provided them with considerable control over committee appointments, which, in turn, allowed them significant control over the legislative business of the House and Senate where committees were crucial in the legislative process. All of this took place in a context in which southern congressional representatives typically demonstrated intense commitment to resisting any federal intrusion into matters of states' rights—typically those matters related to the protection of the institution of segregation—in the face of relative indifference on the part of nonsouthern members of Congress more broadly.

In doing so the southern contingent in Congress had three policy mechanisms at its disposal to ensure that federal policies would not intrude on the social organization of the South (see Katznelson 2005; Lieberman 1998). The first was the ability to design policy in a race-laden, if not explicitly racially based, manner to exclude most African Americans. As outlined more fully below, this was the case with old-age pensions under Social Security that excluded farm laborers and domestic servants from coverage—effectively excluding a large proportion of African Americans in the South. Alternatively, where African Americans were to be included in a program, the southern congressional contingent could apply pressure to leave the administration of the program to the state and local levels. This was the model that social assistance under Aid to Dependent Children (ADC) would adopt by which payments to families with children would be administered by state and local officials—often under starkly discriminatory circumstances. Finally, the southern bloc could also prevent the inclusion of antidiscrimination provisions in legislation.

These patterns, which allowed southern congressional representatives to exercise a veto over national legislation, led to a series of peculiar coalitions as the support of the South was required to pass any national legislation. Northern labor allied itself within the Democratic Party with the South in support of expansive social policies designed, however, to ensure they would not encroach upon the racial status quo of the South. In this context racial discrimination and segregation remained the official and unofficial policy of the federal government until the late 1940s (see King 1995).

Segregation in Health Services

In the general context of legally enforced racial segregation, the provision of health services throughout the United States was deeply marked by racial segregation, which existed in various forms well into the postwar period.[1] In certain geographical areas and especially the North, segregation existed in only limited aspects of heath service provision. In others, especially the South, segregation existed in all aspects of health service provision.

Of the multiple dimensions of health services segregation, the most obvious was the segregation of patients through either the segregation of entire institutions or, alternatively, the segregation of patients within a given institution. While segregated facilities were separate, they were not as a rule equal:

> Hospitals that cared solely for black persons were inferior to those that care for white persons, and facilities that were designated for black persons in mixed-race hospitals included and were sometimes limited to a basement, attic or separate building behind the main hospital. Consequently, equality in health care remained an elusive dream for black people (Reynolds 1997b, 898).

Segregation of hospitals could be a matter of formal policy, as was typically the case in the South, or, alternatively, it could occur as the extension of residential segregation as tended to be the case in the North. By 1957, only 13 percent of general hospitals in northern states continued to have formal discriminatory admissions practices. Conversely, only 10 percent of southern hospitals had formal policies of racial integration. In four states (Arkansas, Georgia, North Carolina, and Texas) there were no integrated general hospitals even as late as 1957 (Cornely 1957, 8–9).

Health services were also segregated by virtue of segregation of medical education, hospital staffs, and professional societies. Medical education historically had been segregated by institution. Initially nine all-black institutions provided training for African American physicians, although, as a result of the reforms wrought by the Flexner Report, by the 1950s only two—Howard and Meharry—survived (Cobb 1957, 3). Approved internships could be completed by African Americans only at ten all-black hospitals. Medical school desegregation in the South only began in 1948, and a decade later roughly half of southern medical schools had begun to accept African American students (Cobb 1957, 7). In some cases integration existed on the level of formal policy but not in practice.[2]

In all southern states African American physicians historically were excluded from county and state medical societies and, by extension, the AMA (Cobb 1957, 3). The first southern medical society to which African Americans were admitted was in Baltimore in 1946 (Journal of the National Medical Association 1960, 199). By 1957 all southern states, with the exception of Louisiana, had taken some step toward the admission of African American physicians although, in some cases such as North Carolina, this was only in the form of limited membership. Patterns of segregation were similar for the nursing profession although integration took place earlier and more smoothly than was the case for physicians.

Hospital staff segregation and segregation of professional societies were often linked. The granting of staff privileges in many hospitals was contingent on membership in the local or state chapter of the AMA—even though in many cases these chapters excluded African Americans. In the South in 1957 only 9 percent of hospitals allowed African American interns and only one-quarter of hospitals had African American staff members, and even in some of these cases, African American physicians were only granted privileges in segregated sections of hospital facilities (Cornely 1957, 9). In instances where nursing staffs were integrated, hospital administrators often remained reluctant to promote African American nurses to positions were they had authority over white nurses. In contrast to the stark North–South differences in the prevalence of mixed-race admissions policies, levels of staff integration in the North were similar to those in the South, with only 13 percent of hospitals accepting African American interns and only one-quarter of hospitals having African American staff members. In some areas of the North such as Chicago, no major hospitals granted staff privileges to African American physicians even in the 1950s (Morris 1960, 211).

Given these practices it is not surprising that challenging hospital segregation would become a central goal of the civil rights movement (Cobb 1953, 438). However, integration in this realm would pose a more serious political challenge than had been the case, for example, in education. First, integration of hospitals faced the challenge posed by the physical nature of the related activities—the general maxim being that integration was easiest for activities in which people are standing, more difficult for activities in which people are sitting, and most difficult in spheres where people are lying down. As a result even in the mid-1960s it was the case that "hospitals remained highly segregated institutions in the sections of the country in which Jim Crow social arrangements lingered, because hospital activities involved intimate body functions in which racial taboos were strongest" (Berkowitz 2003, 146). Moreover, hospital integration required not only exposing patients but also their families to an integrated environment.

Integration in hospitals also faced obstacles created by irrational but potent anxieties regarding medical treatment in an integrated setting. The types of fears raised by integration in health services were embodied most powerfully in the segregation of blood supplies. Under the policies of the American Armed Forces, African Americans were banned from donating blood to the American Red Cross in 1941. In early 1942 the Red Cross lifted the ban under the requirement that African American blood be labeled and segregated from "white blood" (Polsky 2002, 180). Under pressure the Red Cross would later abandon the blood segregation policy in 1950 (NAACP 1950). However, when it did so, various states (such as Louisiana and Arkansas) would enforce the continued segregation of the blood supply through enactment of their own blood segregation laws, which were in effect into the late 1950s.[3]

The degree of racial bias in the provision of health services and the health service professions is disturbingly evident in the horrific Tuskegee syphilis experiment. Over a forty-year period from the 1930s to the 1970s, nearly four hundred African American males with tertiary syphilis were observed by U.S. Public Health Service officials to determine the nature of complications arising from the late stages of the disease. Many of the subjects were unaware that they had syphilis and were offered no treatment for the disease (Jones 1993). This example highlights the depth to which segregation had penetrated health services and is emblematic of the deeply racialized context in which public health insurance reform took place.

Public Health Insurance Initiatives in the United States, 1910–20

Significant efforts at health insurance reform were widespread through the Progressive Era to the end of World War I. At the peak of the Progressive Era, the 1912 presidential campaign of Theodore Roosevelt under the banner of the Progressive Party included, as a central plank in its platform, support for national health insurance (Starr 1982, 243). With Woodrow Wilson's victory, however, reform at the national level would be delayed, and the focus of health insurance reformers turned to the state level.

Serious attempts at health insurance reform subsequently emerged in at least a dozen states (including the most populous such as New York and California) between 1915 and 1919 though none was successful (Walker 1969, 298–300). Reform in California required a ballot initiative for a constitutional amendment, held in 1918, in which the initiative was defeated. Other states considered compulsory insurance directly. In 1916 New York, Massachusetts, and New Jersey each introduced bills for compulsory health insurance based on a standard bill prepared by the American Association for Labor Legislation (AALL). Another twelve states considered the issue in the following year. While most of these state-level proposals never made it out of their respective legislative committees, two such bills were passed by the state senate of New York only to be subsequently defeated in the assembly (Walker 1969, 298).

As would be the case with numerous later attempts at reform, observers would attribute the defeat of public health insurance reform in this period to the role of powerful interest groups—especially organized medicine—operating in the context of highly fragmented political institutions (Starr 1982, 252). Organized medicine, which had been in favor of national health insurance and would remain formally so until the AMA officially reversed its position in 1920, did indeed become increasingly resistant to such schemes. In the context of world war, opposition groups including organized medicine capitalized on anti-German sentiment by arguing that social insurance was a German idea—"a Prussian menace inconsistent with American values" (Starr 1982, 252).

To some significant degree these attempts failed—not primarily because they garnered considerable interest group opposition—but because, in the context of the war, they failed to generate sufficient public interest:

> Certainly the well-organized forces of the opposition greatly harmed the movement. But what assured its defeat was its failure to capture the public imagination. . . . The public did not respond. Somehow, interest never penetrated to the level of the workingman. It remained an intellectual's movement. Without popular backing, the reformers could not overcome either the effects of preoccupation with the war or the well-organized campaign of the "United Front." The movement was forgotten (Walker 1969, 303–4).

Health insurance reform would lie dormant in the American states until the early 1930s.

National Health Insurance and the New Deal

In a special presidential message Franklin D. Roosevelt, in response to conditions created by the Great Depression, announced his intention to appoint the Committee on Economic Security (CES). The committee was directed to study the issue of social insurance, and Roosevelt made a specific commitment to proposals dealing with the problems of unemployment and old age (Witte 1963, 6–7). While the message directed the CES to study the issue of health insurance, health insurance was never seriously considered as a central element of Roosevelt's New Deal. Health services simply were not a priority of the administration and were not at the top of the list of social ills that had been so severely exacerbated by the Depression. The main problem caused by the Depression, in the eyes of policymakers, was loss of income (or savings), and the main policy responses would be geared to addressing these problems and, especially, buoying consumer demand.[4]

The potential effect of proposed New Deal arrangements on the racial structure in the South was a central point of concern for southern political leaders, and getting the package through Congress required a number of compromises to ensure that the federal initiative would pose as minimal a threat as possible to the racial status quo in the South. One central compromise was that agricultural and domestic workers, who composed a large proportion of the southern African American workforce, be excluded from eligibility for contributory pensions. A second compromise was that social assistance and unemployment insurance be administered by the states, which would determine eligibility and levels of benefits (Quadagno 1988; Starr 1982, 269). These two compromises would later contribute significantly in shaping the politics of health insurance reform. In addition, a requirement in the old-age assistance program (federal assistance for state programs for the needy aged) that programs provide a "reasonable subsistence compatible with decency and health" was removed because southern congressional leaders were concerned that the requirement could be used to force states to provide higher benefits to African Americans than they otherwise would—potentially challenging the basis of the southern sharecropper economy.

For its part, had health insurance been included in this package it would have undoubtedly reflected a similar type of compromise. For example, the system of health insurance proposed by the CES was a "permissive" program under which states would receive a federal subsidy if they were to meet certain basic federal safeguards: "Our design for health insurance leaves to the States the initiative in creating systems of insurance. The Federal Government would undertake to lay down general safeguards and to give financial aid to the States." Presaging the rationale of later proposals posed as alternatives to a national program of health insurance, "Our proposals . . . are designed to meet the needs of the American people under the conditions which exist in our States and local communities" (Witte 1963, 210). Moreover, none of the health provisions that were included in the New Deal legislation including federal funding for maternal and infant care, aid for dependent children, or funding for state medical assistance for the blind contained antidiscrimination provisions (Byrd and Clayton 2002, 142).

The acceptance of racial segregation in health services by the federal government was strikingly illustrated by the degree of segregation existing in the Veterans Administration system. From its beginning in 1921 the Veterans Bureau (which was to become the Veterans Administration in 1930) established segregated health services. Protests by the black medical establishment as early as the 1920s had secured African American staffing of Veterans Bureau hospitals for black veterans (such as the facility at Tuskegee) but were not able to forestall institutional segregation (Byrd and Clayton 2002, 129; Morais 1967, 98, 113–15). In fact there was concern among African American leaders in the early 1930s that the VA threatened to extend segregation to "Northern areas such as New York City where officially segregated governmental hospital facilities did not exist" although resistance from the black health care civil rights movement forestalled such developments (Byrd and Clayton 2002, 186). As of 1947, 24 of 127 VA hospitals had separate wards for black patients and 19 hospitals, all in the South, refused to admit blacks except in case of emergency (Byrd and Clayton 2002, 257–58). Federal government treatment of African American veterans provides no reason to believe that it would have adopted a different approach in regard to health services provided under national health insurance.

Even in the mid-1940s as the federal government crafted a GI bill of rights "the Veterans Administration (whose hospitals and housing were racially segregated) knew that legislation for veterans had to pass through southern hands and garner southern backing in Congress. To cultivate this support, they made clear that they were disinclined to challenge the region's race relations and enforce equal treatment for all veterans" (Katznelson 2005, 123). The VA's acceptance of segregation would continue until, following the integration of the armed forces two years earlier, southern VA hospitals began to integrate black patients "under pressure of a directive from the VA's chief medical administrator" beginning in 1950 (Beardsley 1987, 258; Byrd and Clayton 2002, 258). It was only as of October 1954, following the Brown decision, that the VA ordered the end of segregation in all VA hospitals (Byrd and Clayton 2002, 258).

Despite its exclusion from the New Deal, health insurance would remain—albeit peripherally—on the political agenda. Three years later the Interdepartmental Committee to Coordinate Health and Welfare Activities made a similar recommendation to that of the CES: federal subsidization of state-operated medicare programs (Starr 1982, 276). In response to the report Roosevelt called a national health conference that supported the committee's recommendations (Starr, 1982, 276). Roosevelt was "enthusiastic" about national health insurance and initially considered making it a central issue in either the 1938 or 1940 elections. Instead, he recommended Congress give the plan "careful study" but did not immediately give support to legislation (Starr 1982, 277).

In 1939 the recommendations were embodied in a bill introduced in Congress by Senator Robert Wagner of New York. Under the Wagner proposal, enactment of health insurance would be the prerogative of each state. Although the bill was "reported to only face minor opposition in the Senate," it never received presidential support (Starr 1982, 277). Senior administration official Arthur Altmeyer was to argue later that had Roosevelt supported the Wagner Bill, it would have passed in Congress. The reasons for waning presidential support, given Roosevelt's initial enthusiasm, are not all that clear. It has been argued that a key element was that the administration, in the wake of the 1938 elections, faced a congressional alliance of conservative Dixiecrats and Republicans that "made any further innovations in social policy extremely difficult" (Starr 1982, 277). In any event, progress stalled, and with the outbreak of World War II, the second wave of national health insurance reform in the United States ended. As had been the case with the first round of reform in the Progressive era, sputtering health insurance reform at the national level would be eclipsed by reform efforts at the state level.

Post–New Deal Health Insurance Reform in the American States

In the fifteen years after 1935 compulsory health insurance bills were introduced in over a dozen states (Anderson 1951, 111). In 1939 four state bills were proposed for non-means-tested public medical care in New York, Oklahoma, and two in Tennessee.[5] In New York the proposal was to make "medical services free to the entire population on the same basis as public education" (Shearon 1940, 34). Bills for providing a state system of compulsory health insurance were proposed in seven states including California, Massachusetts, New York, Pennsylvania, Rhode Island, and Wisconsin (Shearon 1940, 35). Ultimately none of these reforms would prove to be successful and either "met open opposition or was allowed to die for lack of support"[6] (Shearon 1940, 34). Health insurance again gained renewed momentum in the early 1940s, and twenty-eight bills were introduced in ten states over the 1939–44 period, which provided for statewide systems of compulsory health insurance.[7] The fate of these proposals reprised the fate of state reform efforts in the Progressive era—a building of momentum that stalled in a context of public indifference and world war (Stucke 1952, 1564).

The most sustained campaign for compulsory public health insurance would take place in California. The earlier debate on health insurance reform in California had led to a referendum on a constitutional amendment (through a ballot proposition) allowing for a state-supported compulsory plan in 1918. Although it attracted national attention, it was defeated. Interest in public health insurance in California reemerged in the wake of the failure at the federal level to include health insurance in the New Deal. The Democratic election platform in 1938 included state health insurance, and, upon election: "The new governor [Olson] proclaimed this plan to be 'central' to his administration" (Mitchell 2002, 11–12).[8] The California Medical Association initially supported medical insurance reform but, in the face of a program that was unlikely to meet the doctors' preferred plan, its position quickly shifted to opposition (Mitchell 2002, 11).

The most important obstacle was the issue of cost and the fiscal challenges for California of going it alone. Despite the fact that Democrats controlled the state legislature, the plan was unable to muster sufficient legislative support primarily due to concerns over cost. There was little reason for state legislators to anticipate federal financial aid, and "had such federal funding been available, perhaps the cost to the state would have been less of an obstacle despite its Depression-era fiscal constraints" (Mitchell 2002, 12). It would be the second of a series of seven defeats for public (or publicly mandated) health insurance in the state of California, with the next three occurring between 1945 and 1948.

In late 1944 California Governor Earl Warren presented another plan for public health insurance.[9] In the ensuing public debate, the medical profession led a high-profile and high-cost public assault on the proposed plan. However, even so, public opinion remained fluid, and "although public opinion was enlisted by both sides, ultimately the matter had to be fought out in the legislature" (Mitchell 2002, 22).[10] The Public Health Committee refused to send the bill to the house floor, and an assembly vote to force the bill to the floor was defeated by one vote in April 1945—at which point, it became clear that the plan was dead (Mitchell 2002, 23). It had been, however, the narrowest of defeats.

Almost immediately Warren proposed a public insurance plan limited to hospital care. This proposal continued to meet strong resistance from physicians as they feared that "hospitals might start to offer (state-subsidized) medical services in competition with doctors" (Mitchell 2002, 24). Again the Public Health Committee refused to send the bill to the house floor. And again an Assembly vote to force the bill to the house floor was narrowly defeated by handful of votes. Despite these failures Warren was comfortably reelected in 1946. With a strong electoral mandate behind him, Warren proposed an even more modest plan in early 1947 covering only catastrophic hospital expenses that again never made it out of committee (Mitchell 2002, 25). It seems very unlikely that Warren would have invested such huge amounts of political capital in public health insurance if success seemed impossible.

The failure of the Warren plan, considering the size and significance of California in the American federal system, has been argued to have had important implications for health care reform in other states: "A success by Warren in California might have sparked liberals in other states to push to emulate the California example. . . . By the same token, defeat of Warren's health plans may have discouraged politicians in other states from proposing similar programs" (Mitchell 2002, 20). Mitchell speculates that the failure of the Warren plan also had crucial implications for federal level reform and, as such, "the turning point in US health care history may well have come before defeat of the Truman proposal and . . . its location may well have been Sacramento in 1945–47, not Washington, DC in 1949" (Mitchell 2002, 30). Mitchell raises a number of interesting speculative questions:

> If Warren had succeeded in enacting a California health plan, would other states have followed? Might the later Truman effort have been devoted to fostering state plans rather than enacting a single national plan? Might the US, in short, have ended up with a system resembling Canada's provincially-operated single-payer arrangements? There are some reasons to think this alternative sequence of events was a possibility (2002, 20).

As will be argued below, this alternate sequence of events seems unlikely. Success at the state level simply was not very likely in the absence of any prospects for federal cost-sharing. By the late 1940s any federal program—whether nationally administered or a federal–state grant-in-aid program—would have faced serious difficulties as a result of the shifting politics of civil rights. At the same time, the failure of reform at the state level reinforced the orientation of reformers toward the federal level—an orientation that, because of the entanglement of public health insurance and the issue of civil rights, ultimately dimmed the prospects for successful reform.

The Canadian Context and Public Health Insurance Initiatives, 1910–40

Echoing health reform initiatives in the United States, two major developments in Canadian health insurance reform would take place in this period: the commitment of the federal Liberal Party under to-be Prime Minister Mackenzie King to national health insurance in 1919 and, more concretely, health insurance reform initiatives in British Columbia.

Health reform debates in Canada in this early period were influenced by the attempts at health insurance reform south of the border highlighting the political and cultural similarities between the two countries. Public health insurance "rumblings" in the United States would have significance for Canadian health care reform, and some of the impetus for early debates on public health insurance in Canada came from the United States (Naylor 1986, 35; Taylor 1990, 38). Public health insurance reformers in Canada would draw inspiration from the AALL. Similarly the CMA would also be influenced by its American counterpart, the AMA. During the early period of AMA support for public health insurance, the CMA was paying close to attention to developments in the United States and the emerging American literature on health insurance (Naylor 1986, 37). Just as the support of organized medicine for public health insurance would wax and wane in the United States, so too would this be the case in Canada. Increasing professional opposition to public health insurance in Canada reflected, in part, the degree to which "Canadian doctors were influenced by the attitudes of their American confreres" (Naylor 1986, 39, 45). During this period AMA leaders would address major Canadian medical societies such as the Ontario Medical Association (OMA) regarding the "evils" of public health insurance (Naylor 1986, 46).

At the same time, these debates took place in a radically different political context. Territorial tensions between the English and French had been woven into the fabric of the Canadian territory following the conquest in 1759 of New France (present-day Québec) by the British—well before Canada even became a country. The British Act of Union of 1840 that united Upper Canada (present-day Ontario) and Lower Canada (present-day Québec) had been proposed by Lord Durham who had been sent to Lower Canada by the British government following rebellions in both Upper Canada and Lower Canada in 1837 and 1838. Describing the situation in Lower Canada where the rebellion had been considerably more serious, Durham noted: "I expected to find a contest between a government and a people: I found two nations warring in the bosom of a single state: I found a struggle, not of principles, but of *races*" (Lambton 1839, emphasis added). Durham's recommendations, which were adopted in the Act of Union, were clearly assimilationist—the war between "races" could be attenuated only by the assimilation of the French into a larger English-dominated polity. This policy of assimilation, however, failed and was replaced by a new vision embodied in the British North America Act, 1867, that created the new country of Canada through the joining of the Province of Canada (Ontario and Québec) with the colonies of Nova Scotia and New Brunswick.

The BNA Act provided constitutional grants of powers to the Dominion (national) government while outlining a range of matters that would be exclusively provincial jurisdiction. This arrangement thus recognized the legitimacy of the French-speaking majority in the new Province of Québec to retain control over various aspects of government crucially related to the protection of the French culture and language within Québec. Notably, the BNA Act would provide the preponderance of jurisdictional authority over health care to the provinces. The broader accommodation would provide the basis for later visions of Canadian confederation as a compact between two founding peoples (English and French) in which each were to be equal partners—a vision that remains evident albeit highly contentious today. The federal solution accommodated but did not resolve English–French tensions, which continued to underlay Canadian political life and which periodically burst onto the political scene with considerable force.

In the United States the increasingly dominant form of social organization in regard to racial minorities was exclusion—especially in the South. African Americans in the South were largely disenfranchised, and they had no access to the levers of political power. Conversely, in Canada, the concentration of the French linguistic minority in the province of Québec meant that they had ready access to crucial levers of political power—especially control of the provincial government. Moreover, because of the geographic concentration of French-speaking voters in Québec, their support was an important element for federal parties in developing and maintaining a national, governing coalition. Finally, as would become evident later, the overlapping of geographical boundaries with ethnolinguistic cleavages would allow for the possibility of secession.

Federal Health Insurance Reform and Territorial Politics in Canada

The first major commitment to national public health insurance in Canada would set a pattern that would mark virtually every major federal government initiative in the field. The federal government would attempt to assert (or reassert) its role in the provision of public health insurance in the wake of a broader crisis involving the flaring of nationalist sentiment in Québec.

Mandatory military service (typically referred to in Canada as conscription) became the most serious flashpoint of linguistic tensions in Canada in both the first and second world wars. Linguistic tensions were already high in the wake of passage of Bill 17 in Ontario in 1912, which restricted the teaching of the French language in that province. Canada's participation in what were seen in Québec to be imperial wars of the British government exacerbated these tensions. In 1917 the Conservative government of Prime Minister Robert Borden passed the Military Service Act implementing a military draft, prompting riots in Québec City in which four people were killed. The Conservative Party's political support in Québec would be destroyed as a result of this crisis in which Québec decisively rejected the federal government's authority in this regard.

It was in this context that the Liberal Party would make a vague commitment in 1919 (in preparing its platform for the 1921 election) to national public health insurance under its new leader, William Lyon Mackenzie King, an industrial relations expert strongly predisposed toward social insurance.[11] Despite this commitment no substantive action would be taken, and little public debate regarding national public health insurance would occur until, as was the case in the United States, health insurance reform arose as an issue in the context of a federal government response to the Great Depression.

As of the early 1920s enthusiasm on the part of Canadian physicians for public insurance was "decidedly absent" (Naylor 1986, 45). However, with the advent of economic depression in the 1930s, concern arose in regard to physician incomes. The CMA, along with provincial medical associations, lobbied for medical relief programs to cover uncompensated care provided to indigents, which had exploded during the Depression (See Naylor 1986, 65–68). The CMA would approach Prime Minister Bennett directly as early as 1933 in this regard although he would maintain that the matter was strictly under provincial purview.[12] Over this period the CMA outlined the terms under which it would support public health insurance including the following: "(a) that the majority of members on health insurance commissions be representatives of organized medicine; (b) that the method of remunerating doctors for their services must be suitable to organized medicine; (c) that the fee schedule be under complete control of organized medicine; and (d) that the system be restricted to those below a certain income level" (Guest 1997, 100; Taylor 1978, 25). Certainly these terms would have met with favor from the AMA and, as discussed earlier, are highly consistent with the proposals of the medical profession in California in the mid-1930s.

Nevertheless, health insurance was not included in the federal government's New Deal. In the final days of the Conservative government in 1935, Bennett introduced his version of a New Deal including provisions for social insurance legislation. Similar to the social insurance components of Roosevelt's New Deal, the package emphasized unemployment insurance and contributory old-age pensions, but Bennett also proposed "health, accident, and sickness insurance" (Guest 1997, 88). Of the series of bills Bennett had proposed to submit to parliament, the only one actually submitted was the Employment and Social Insurance Act of 1935, which dealt almost exclusively with the issue of unemployment. Similar to Roosevelt's final package, the new administrative commission (similar to the Social Security Administration in the New Deal package) was given a mandate only to study medical and hospital care insurance (Taylor 1990, 44). As was the case in the United States, health insurance would not be included in the Canadian New Deal, and further attempts at health insurance reform would have to wait until after World War II.

Public Health Insurance Reform in British Columbia

Following the initial public discussions on the matter in the early 1920s, serious efforts at public health insurance reform would be undertaken in British Columbia in the mid-1930s at the same time that major efforts at reform were being undertaken in California. As in California, the reforms would initially be accepted and later rejected by the medical profession, and both sets of reforms would meet business opposition. While both of these factors were important, more broadly, the main impediment to the BC initiatives was, as had been the case in California, that "British Columbia was acting alone" (Taylor 1990, 32). The similar outcomes in British Columbia and California would highlight not differences in institutional design (for example, separation of powers versus fusion of powers) but, rather, institutional similarities—the difficulty in both countries of undertaking provincial and state reforms in the absence of federal support.

The BC initiative began in 1919 when a demand in the BC legislature for the government to express its policy on the issue of public health insurance resulted in the striking of a royal commission of inquiry. Despite the fact that public health insurance reform was already dead in most of the American states where reform efforts had taken place, the commission was clearly very aware of attempts at reform in the United States and included reports as well as draft legislation from several American states (Taylor 1990, 38). The commission recommended the adoption of a provincial system of health insurance although the report was not released and the recommendation was never implemented.[13] The rationale offered by the BC premier was that health insurance was a federal concern (according to a recently concluded federal–provincial conference); instead, he called on the federal government to implement a scheme (Naylor 1986, 44). Despite this brief flicker health insurance reform in the Canadian provinces, as in the U.S. states, would wait over decade before being reignited.

Despite the fact that nearly all federal and provincial governments studied the issue of health care in the 1920s and 1930s, major attempts at reform took place only at the provincial level in British Columbia and Alberta where public health insurance legislation was passed (but not implemented) in 1936 and 1937, respectively.[14] In British Columbia a second royal commission on health insurance had been struck in 1929. Its report of 1932 recommended a compulsory plan for all employed persons (and their dependents) up to an income limit ($2,400 per year) above which the plan would be voluntary. Following the commission recommendations very closely, legislation was introduced in March 1935. Benefits would include "medical and hospital care and, as financial conditions permitted, drugs, diagnostic services, home nursing care and sickness cash benefits"[15] (Taylor 1990, 40–41).

Despite the fact that the CMA was not, in principle, opposed to public health insurance (although it had issued a set of principles to which any public plan would have to conform in order to garner CMA support), the British Columbia College of Physicians and Surgeons was "unanimously and unalterably" opposed.[16] The physicians would dress up their opposition to the proposals in various guises (most notably that the later proposals did not adequately cover low-income groups); however, they were undoubtedly concerned over the degree to which the proposed administrative commission posed a threat to professional autonomy as well as, most important, over "modes and amounts of remuneration" (Naylor 1986, 87).

As had been the case in numerous American states, physician opposition was buttressed by the opposition of the British Columbia Manufacturer's Association, which was concerned about the impact of additional taxation on mining and lumber exports (Taylor 1990, 41; Naylor 1986, 77). A report for the Royal Commission on Dominion–Provincial relations, discussed more fully below, would conclude that jurisdiction over social insurance "tends to militate against the introduction of social insurance because any given province is afraid that if it takes the lead it will penalize its own industry in competition with that of other provinces" (Grauer 1939, 55). For the same reasons, organized labor, including the British Columbia Loggers Association, was also opposed: "Health Insurance should not be established in British Columbia until it becomes a national policy all over Canada, in order that the highly protected industries of eastern Canada should be compelled to contribute as well as the basic industries of British Columbia, which do not benefit by protective tariffs but must sell their products in the open markets of the world" (*Canadian Medical Association Journal* 1936, 232). This position reflected a widespread belief that social insurance, in raising the prices of manufactured goods that were labor intensive, was particularly injurious to the competitiveness of primary industries that suffered higher input prices as a result yet, at the same time, remained price takers on the world market (Grauer 1939, 57). The concentration of manufacturing industries in central Canada and primary industry in the Canadian hinterland thus transformed this issue of social policy into a territorial issue involving concerns of inter-regional equity and clearly signaled the need for federal intervention.

Despite this concerted opposition, an amended bill (which dropped the provision that the government would pay the premiums for low-income people) was reintroduced in March 1936 and passed (Taylor 1990, 42). Registration of employers was completed, enrollment of employees was well under way, and the government announced that the program coverage would be effective in early 1937. However, resistance from the medical profession would ultimately force the government to delay: "Meanwhile, negotiations with the profession were deadlocked, the college announcing on February 1 that the profession, by an almost unanimous vote in a referendum, refused to work under the program. Finally, it became clear that the project was just too much . . . the premier . . . announce[d] on February 9 that the program would be postponed until after an election, which he later called for June 2, 1937" (Taylor 1990, 42). The election included a referendum question on the issue of comprehensive health insurance. The vote was close, with 56 percent voting in favor and 44 percent opposing—much closer than reformers had anticipated (Taylor 1990, 42). Despite the fact that the government was returned with an overwhelming, if somewhat diminished, majority with double the seats of the combined opposition and a favorable majority vote in the referendum, it did not move forward with the plan.

The response of the British Columbia Medical Association (BCMA), similar to responses of medical associations in the American states, was to aggressively enter the voluntary health insurance arena: "The most aggressive action to put the profession into the health insurance business was that of the British Columbia Medical Association (BCMA), still shaken from its bitter, though successful, battle against the British Columbia government's proposed program from 1934 to 1937. Now keenly aware of the aroused public opinion favoring health insurance, the BCMA decided to develop an organization that would sell a service contract to employee groups through their employer, who would be required to contribute a minimum of 50 percent of the premium" (Taylor 1990, 62). The plan was highly successful, and "by the midforties BCMSA enrollment reached over one-quarter million subscribers" (Taylor 1990, 63). However, as discussed more fully below, this would not forestall a provincial plan for compulsory hospital insurance in the late 1940s.

Health insurance proposals also emerged in this period in Alberta. The United Farmers of Alberta (UFA) endorsed health insurance in the 1921 election, which it won (Taylor 1990, 43). The government, however, did not move on the issue of health insurance. The 1927 UFA party convention passed a resolution in favor of state medical services. The proposed program was premised on a populist philosophical base and was intended to weaken the overwhelming control of medical practice by medical professionals who, in the words of the resolution, were inclined to put self-interest before the welfare of the patient (Naylor 1986, 31). A legislative committee was later established to study the issue, which it did from 1929 to 1932 when a royal commission was set up. The commission reported in 1934, and legislation was passed a year later recommending the further development of municipal doctor and hospital plans to be followed, at a later date, by provincial health insurance (Taylor 1990, 43). Shortly after the legislation was passed, the government was defeated in a general election, and no action was taken on the 1935 health insurance legislation (Taylor 1990, 43).

Conclusions

Rather than emphasizing differences between the two countries, these early efforts at reform emphasize similarities in political culture and the institutional effects of federalism. The political cultures of the two countries were not sufficiently distinct to be reflected in fundamental differences in the main policy options being considered or in significant differences in the tenor and language of health reform debates. The opposition of the medical profession was as vociferous in British Columbia as it was in the American states, raising doubts about claims that the position of the medical profession in the two countries reflected broader differences in political culture (Tuohy 1999). Early attempts at health insurance reform were not undertaken by governments controlled by social democratic parties in British Columbia or Alberta, raising doubts about claims that health insurance reform in Canada was the result of an institutional configuration that was more likely to give rise to social democratic parties at the provincial level (Maioni 1998). Finally, institutional differences between the American states and Canadian provinces, such as the separation versus fusion of powers systems, in the face of determined efforts at reform in both California and British Columbia, did not translate into different outcomes.

Rather, the comparable outcomes in the two countries in this period emphasize an important institutional similarity between them—the degree to which their federal systems augured against health insurance reform by individual states and provinces. In both countries the main obstacle to the most vigorous attempts at reform stemmed from the fact of the state (California) or province (British Columbia) "going it alone" in its attempts to implement public health insurance. Successful reform would require the involvement of the federal government.

As argued below later attempts at federal reform would also result in similar outcomes in both countries. It was in this later period that the politics of health insurance reform would become fully bound up in the differences in context created by the politics of race and territorial integration outlined in this chapter. Federal involvement in public health insurance in both countries would, at least initially, be forestalled by the opposition of sectional interests in the South and in Québec, which would use crucial levers of institutional power to successfully oppose national programs of public health insurance threatening to disrupt established social relations in those regions. The seeds of distinct trajectories of development in the United States and Canada, however, would be sown as the politics of public health insurance would become increasingly enmeshed with the politics of race in the former and the politics of territorial integration in the latter.

PART II

Public Health Insurance in the United States

CHAPTER THREE

Failure of Reform in the Truman Era, 1943–52

I don't see anything socialistic about that [compulsory health insurance]. It's absolutely necessary, and I'm going to fight for it until I die.

Harry S. Truman, President

The greatest of all discriminatory evils [is the] differential treatment toward African Americans with respect to hospital facilities.

W. Montague Cobb, National Medical Association

THE ISSUE OF national health insurance emerged again on the political agenda in the United States as World War II drew to a close. This time, however, debates over health insurance were marked by two important shifts in context. First, the most visible shift from the perspective of health insurance reformers was the winning of presidential support for the cause of national health insurance, with President Roosevelt giving reform leaders private assurances of his support (Poen 1979, 29). In January 1944 Roosevelt asked Congress to affirm an economic bill of rights including "the right to adequate medical care," which did not, however, pass before Roosevelt's death. Upon Roosevelt's death, the issue was left to his successor, Harry S. Truman, who demonstrated an even more forceful commitment to national health insurance. The second major shift was the changing context resulting from the politics of civil rights and the resulting federal shift away from a formal policy of segregation in the postwar period.

Given the coincidence of these two shifts, it is not surprising that in the Truman era the politics of national public health insurance and the politics of race became inextricably interwoven: the administration explicitly linked its policies on health insurance and its antisegregation program; support and opposition to national compulsory health insurance was drawn along racial as well as segregationist/integrationist lines; and opposition to national compulsory health insurance was framed in ways that both explicitly and inadvertently raised issues relating to segregation.

Over the seven years from 1945 to 1952, a number of bills providing for national public health insurance were presented to Congress with presidential support. None, however, passed, and the only significant health legislation adopted during President Truman's tenure provided federal cost-sharing for hospital construction. Examinations of public health insurance reform in this period make reference to various explanatory factors including, most notably, the opposition of powerful interest groups such as the AMA, the institutional fragmentation of the American political system, and the role of voluntary insurance in limiting the political prospects for public health insurance. Each of these factors had an important impact on the outcome of national health insurance debates in this period. The dynamics generated by the politics of race, however, were a crucial element contributing to the demise of national public health insurance in this period.

The Politics of Race and the Failure of National Health Insurance, 1945–52

The introduction of the first of a long series of national health insurance bills sponsored by Senator Robert Wagner of New York, Senator James Murray of Montana, and Representative John Dingell of Michigan in 1943 marked the revival of the debate over national health insurance. The bill provided for a comprehensive, public, prepaid, medical care plan (Poen 1979, 31). The plan provided both physician care (on a scheduled fee-for-service basis) and limited hospital care (up to sixty days per year) funded through payroll taxes.[1] Whereas earlier proposals had been for a federal–state permissive program, the new proposals were for a straight federal program.[2]

National health insurance garnered the support of President Truman in 1945, and health security quickly moved to the top of Truman's postwar domestic reform priorities (Poen 1979, 61). The first explicit presidential support for a program of national health insurance was embodied in Truman's special message to Congress in November 1945. The resulting legislation, S. 1606, was yet another version of the Wagner–Murray–Dingell bill and provided for national compulsory health insurance administered by the federal government, grants-in-aid to the states (for health services for the needy, public health services, maternal and child health services, and hospital construction) as well as grants in aid to nonprofit institutions for medical research and education (*Congressional Record* 1945, 10790).Of these various proposals, the only legislation relating to health that was ultimately successful was the Hill–Burton Act of 1946 that provided federal funding for hospital construction. Not only was the Hill–Burton program a federal–state permissive program (states were not required to participate) but it also explicitly included a separate-but-equal provision directly in the legislation. Facilities built using federal funds could be racially segregated as long as the overall result did not lead to health services being inequitably distributed on the basis of race.

Hill–Burton could be seen as a compromise that allowed for federal aid in the provision of health services while forestalling incursions into areas deemed to be matters of "states' rights" that might challenge the racial status quo. As national compulsory health insurance stalled in the late 1940s, the Hill–Burton hospital construction program was repeatedly enriched and liberalized. The basic compromise Hill–Burton entailed endured until the early 1960s when it was challenged not only in Congress but also, decisively, in the courts. In retrospect the Hill–Burton Act appears to have defined the political limits of federal intrusion in the health field in this period—limits upon which more ambitious efforts at reform would founder.

The Administration's Strategy for National Health Insurance

Despite the earlier failure to advance national compulsory health insurance, Truman again appealed to Congress in May 1947. In this Congress, however, the politics of health insurance became even more seriously complicated by Truman's stance on civil rights. The Truman administration's civil rights initiative and national health insurance plan were linked not only by the timing of their presentation to Congress but also through explicit calls by senior administration officials for the racial integration of hospitals and having a high-profile integrationist official, Oscar Ewing, spearhead the administration's drive for national compulsory health insurance.

National Health Insurance and Civil Rights

In contrast to the first version of the national health insurance bill (S. 1606), the revised version introduced in 1947 (S. 1320) proposed state, rather than federal, administration. This change was intended to address one of the central stumbling blocks to congressional adoption of S. 1606—the issue of states' rights (*Congressional Record* 1947, 5519). At the same time, however, a prohibition against racial discrimination in the provision of health services was included—a provision that would be carried over into subsequent versions of the national health insurance bill. The 1947 bill, S. 1320, section 255, read as follows: "In carrying out the provisions of this title, there shall be no discrimination on account of race, creed, or color. Personal health services shall be made available as benefits to all eligible individuals, and all persons qualified . . . to furnish or provide such services shall be permitted to do so" (U.S. Senate, Committee on Labor and Public Welfare, Subcommittee on Health 1947, 28). The prohibition was reproduced as section 755 in S. 1679 in 1949 (U.S. Senate, Committee on Labor and Public Welfare, Subcommittee on Health Legislation 1949, 71).

In her book examining the failed development of national health insurance, Quadagno asserts: "The bill included a ban on racial discrimination in health care but made a concession to the South. Southern states would be allowed to provide 'separate facilities for persons of different race or color' as long as they were of 'equal' quality to white facilities" (2005, 34). Quadagno references an editorial in the *Journal of the American Medical Association* as the sole support for this claim. The editorial refers only, however, to the bill's provision for separate-but-equal facilities for medical education—not for the provision of health services (1949, 112).

In June 1947 Truman became the first president to address the National Association for the Advancement of Colored People (NAACP)—a highly publicized event in which Truman addressed a crowd of ten thousand people from the steps of the Lincoln Memorial (McCullough 1992, 569–70). Truman stated that "there is no justifiable reason for discrimination" on the basis of race or color. He argued that the enjoyment of certain basic rights, including among other things the right to "adequate medical care," be enjoyed "on equal terms . . . by every citizen" (1947).

The implications of federal involvement in health insurance for racial segregation in health services were highlighted by the report of the President's Committee on Civil Rights (PCCR) later that year. Among a wide range of recommendations, two were especially critical to the issue of health care. First, in an effort to "eliminate segregation from American life," the report recommended that federal grants-in-aid (to both public and private agencies regardless of purpose) be conditional on the absence of any racial discrimination. Second, the report recommended that all states enact "fair health practice statutes forbidding discrimination and segregation . . . in the operation of public or private health facilities." These recommendations contributed to firmly establishing a link in public debates between federal involvement in the health field and the issue of segregation in health services. The report received strong presidential endorsement, with Truman urging all Americans to read it and claiming that the report could serve as "an American charter of human freedom in our time" (McCoy and Ruetten 1973, 86).

The link between civil rights and health insurance was reinforced by the State of the Union address of 1948 in which Truman outlined two major goals: securing civil rights and developing human resources—primarily through the adoption of compulsory health insurance. While the antisegregation plank of the Truman program touched on a wide number of areas, including segregation in the armed forces, schools, and private accommodations and transportation, it was believed that it would also mandate desegregation of hospitals (*Congressional Record* 1948, A2338). In regard to strengthening human resources, the most important issue, according to the president, was health care, which demanded a national health program, the heart of which "must be a national system of payment for medical care based . . . on insurance principles" (*Congressional Record* 1948, 33).

The political fates of the two programs were closely intertwined. At the Democratic convention in the summer of 1948, a compromise position on civil rights was adopted in an attempt to avoid an open split with the southern faction of the party. In this compromise, the platform committee proposed a weakened civil rights plank. At the same time, national health insurance, which had been included in the initial drafts of the platform, was removed from the program entirely (Poen 1979, 24). Nevertheless, a serious rift in the party emerged when debate on the civil rights plank was forced onto the convention floor. As a result a contingent of southern Democrats broke from the party. In the wake of the rupture a strong civil rights plank was reinserted into the Democratic platform and Truman recommitted himself, in his nomination speech, to national health insurance. Truman called the Eightieth Congress back for a special session in which he asked for the passage of both national compulsory health insurance and his civil rights legislation. Neither package was passed. Truman then made both civil rights and national health insurance central issues in his bid for reelection in 1948, and his surprise victory gave renewed impetus to both causes.

Following Truman's victory national health insurance continued to face fierce opposition from various quarters including, most notably, from southern congressional representatives and the AMA. Various compromises might have been possible, including plans that would have attracted southern congressional support, but for its part the White House gave no indication of any inclination to compromise (Starr 1982, 285; Poen 1979, 167). Doing so would have required compromise not only over the terms of health insurance per se but over the degree to which federal involvement could accommodate segregation in health services and facilities—a much more intractable political problem considering Truman's reliance on the African American vote in 1948 and continuing Democratic aspirations to court the African American vote in the midterm congressional elections of 1950. The first thing mentioned by a "high-ranking Democrat" asked to sum up the achievements of the Eighty-first Congress was that "we haven't lost a Negro vote" (Albright 1949).

The Federal Security Administration and Oscar Ewing

A direct link between civil rights and federal intervention in health services was clearly drawn by senior officials in the Truman administration—most notably, Oscar Ewing, the Federal Security administrator from 1947 to 1952. In January of 1948 Ewing's report *The Nation's Health: A Report to the President* spoke directly to the issue of segregation in health services, noting that "millions of our people are unable to use the hospitals that exist either because they lack the money to pay for services, or because discrimination or segregation closes the doors against them."[3] Ewing called for medical services to be provided to everyone "without regard to his race or religion, the color of his skin, his place of national origin or the place he lives in our land" (1948, 53, 35). As outlined in the report, "We can no longer tolerate in our society a system of medical care under which Negro physicians and Negro patients are discriminated against. . . . There should be no racial barriers in the provision of adequate medical care" (1948, 41). Thus, the report recommended that the federal government provide grants of up to 40 percent of maintenance costs of hospitals in selected low-income areas on the proviso that all staffing be undertaken without racial discrimination (1948, 61). The report received widespread news coverage and was seen as underpinning the administration's national health insurance strategy.

In keeping with the report's recommendations, Ewing personally addressed a number of events (including meetings of various African American organizations) calling for integration both in hospital staffing and in the treatment of patients (*New York Times* [NYT] 1949b, 1949i). Ewing also publicly favored withholding federal funds "wherever policies of 'discrimination' were in force" (NYT 1949b). Moreover, Ewing himself was a high-profile, committed integrationist. He was singularly responsible for a highly publicized move to desegregate the intern program at Gallinger Hospital in Washington, D.C. (NYT 1949f). Furthermore, Ewing received media comment for appointing an African American woman as his own special assistant (Fleeson 1949). Had Truman wished to downplay the link between civil rights and national health insurance, he would have been well advised to have chosen almost anyone other than Ewing as FSA administrator.

Truman's choice of Ewing ultimately had important implications for his attempts at organizational reform of the administration. Truman's Reorganization Plan No. 1 of 1949, which would have elevated the FSA to departmental status, was initially reported in the *Washington Post* to be likely to pass "without delay or serious opposition" (Meyer 1949). Instead, the ensuing vitriolic debate focused to a large degree on Ewing, who was widely expected to become the first secretary of the new department (Meyer 1949; Spargo 1949). In the words of Senator Hubert Humphrey, the "amazing bitterness of this campaign against Oscar Ewing" was "baffling" (*Congressional Record* 1949, 11130).

The opposition to Ewing was obviously not based primarily on his support of health insurance. Various observers felt that it was reasonable to expect that anyone appointed by President Truman to be the secretary of a new department (whether a combined department of health, welfare, and education as was proposed in Reorganization Plan No. 1 or a separate Department of Health as demanded by the AMA) would support the president's national compulsory health insurance plan (Senate Committee on Expenditures in the Executive Departments 1949, 67). Thus, explaining opposition to the reorganization on the basis that the director would be in favor of national health insurance (or, as was repeatedly claimed in committee hearings, that cabinet status would provide greater ability for the director to push for national health insurance) falls flat. In terms of congressional opposition, senior Republicans such as Taft and southern Democrats such as Fulbright had themselves proposed, prior to Ewing's tenure, a reorganization plan similar to the one they so vigorously opposed in 1949.

The stridency of the opposition to Ewing is more easily explained as a reaction to his stand on racial integration of hospitals and health services. The *Washington Daily News* reported that, while the AMA opposed Ewing's support of compulsory health insurance, the opposition in Congress was the result of "Dixiecrats tak[ing] a dim view of his championship of civil rights with the stress he places on Negroes" (*Congressional Record* 1949, 11370). A news article entered in the *Congressional Record* quotes an unnamed southern senator: "I realize that Jack Ewing is no Communist. . . . I also understand the political wisdom of his fight for Negro rights. But I'll be darned if I'm going back home and explain all that. I'll just vote to kill the plan" (*Congressional Record* 1949, 11370). Twenty of the twenty-three Democrats who joined the Republicans to defeat the plan in the Senate were from southern states (Knowless 1949; Spargo 1949). A renewed reorganization attempt in 1950 was defeated in the House with the support of every single southern Democrat. Thus the battle lines over the reorganization plan mirrored those drawn in national health insurance and civil rights.

The Racial Cast of Support and Opposition to National Compulsory Health Insurance

Support and opposition to national compulsory health insurance fell along racial as well as segregationist/antisegregationist lines—suggestive of the link between national public health insurance and civil rights. On the one side the AMA and southern Democrats shared a natural affinity in their opposition to national health insurance. On the other side the NAACP and National Medical Association (NMA) publicly provided strong support for the Truman health insurance plans.

The American Medical Association

The most visible opposition to national compulsory health insurance came from organized medicine under the leadership of the AMA—itself a highly segregated organization. As a result of the AMA's federal structure, state medical societies controlled membership in the national organization (NYT 1949h). The result was that "in the 17 southern States and the District of Columbia, colored physicians are excluded from membership in county and State medical societies" (U.S. Senate Committee, Subcommittee on Health 1947, 1094). State medical societies also were directly involved in hospital staff segregation because state medical society membership was usually required to obtain hospital privileges. The NAACP medical representative, W. Montague Cobb, noted in congressional hearings, "An extension of the exclusion of colored physicians from medical societies is their exclusion from hospital staffs both public and private. This obtains with a few exceptions not only in the South but in the great urban centers of the North and West" (U.S. Senate, Subcommittee on Health 1947, 1094). While the AMA officially supported local control over the issue of staff integration, it also officially opposed any use of federal funds to promote the racial integration of hospital staffs (U.S. House 1946, 103).

Segregation at the state level was mirrored at the national level. The AMA House of Delegates remained "lily-white" until 1949 with only token African American representation thereafter. Thus it is not surprising that there was little pressure from the national level on state societies to end segregationist practices. The segregation of the medical profession into the all-white AMA and all-black National Medical Association removed the voice of African American physicians (who were significantly more disposed to favor national health insurance) from the internal debate within the AMA over health insurance. This further isolated white physicians inside the AMA who were supportive of national health insurance. Racial segregation of the medical profession thus reinforced professional opposition to national health insurance.

This is not to argue that AMA opposition to compulsory health insurance was primarily related to its implications for segregation in health services. Clearly it was not. However, as argued above, the racial segregation the AMA practiced reinforced its opposition to compulsory health insurance. Further, as discussed more fully below, AMA support for segregation contributed to undermining the possibilities for various compromise measures that might have provided a basis for the emergence of national health insurance. Finally, AMA support of segregation underpinned the affinity between the AMA and southern elected representatives who formed the bedrock of congressional opposition to national health insurance.

Congressional Representatives of the Southern States

Southern representatives were a critical component of the opposition coalition in Congress. Of course, the southern congressional caucus was not a monolithic group and included representatives of a range of positions, including "naked and strident racists like Theodore Bilbo and 'Cotton Ed' Smith, urbane and publicly moderate guardians of segregation like Richard Russell, and expert nonracist liberals like Claude Pepper and Lyndon Johnson." Nevertheless, what was key was that "when engaged in the politics of representation outside the region, virtually all the South's members of Congress stood together to preserve the basic contours of the region's racial regime. This was the premise of southern representation and accounted for its survival" (Katznelson 2005, 18, 20).

The southern position on federal aid was paradoxical (Katznelson 2005, 40). On the one hand, southern states were poor and thus desperately needed the financial aid that federal programs could provide. On the other hand, federal intervention posed the risk of federal interference in matters of "state's rights"—a term often used in the South to refer to the ability of state governments to maintain legalized segregation. Thus, southern representatives did not oppose all federal involvement in health services. Most notably they had not used their congressional power to block the Hill–Burton Act to provide federal funding for hospital construction. The quid pro quo for southern support was the explicit provision in the Hill–Burton program allowing for the construction of segregated hospitals using federal funds. Such a compromise on national health insurance, however, was not politically viable for Truman.

The South was generally resistant to federal incursions in policy fields that appeared likely to challenge the racial status quo. For example, proposals for federal aid for education met strong resistance on the basis that federal aid would lead to federal interference in school segregation (*Congressional Record* 1949, 3929). The sentiment in the Upper South, as reported by the *New York Times,* was that "Federal aid would essentially mean Federal control" and that "inevitably this would mean an assault against the South's segregated school system." Not surprisingly, the same article reports that "equally sharp feeling developed over the Federal health bill" (NYT 1949i).

National Association for the Advancement of Colored People and the National Medical Association

On the other side of the debate, prominent African American organizations such as the NAACP and NMA supported national compulsory health insurance. This support demonstrated the race-specific implications of national health insurance. It also contributed to shaping the politics of national health insurance. The NAACP publicly and officially supported all three versions of the national health insurance plan (S. 1606, S. 1320, and S. 1679) as well as Reorganization Plan No. 1 of 1949 (U.S. Senate, Committee on Expenditures in the Executive Departments 1949, 136; Loftus 1949). The NAACP's 1947 national convention, which Truman addressed, adopted a resolution in favor of national health insurance (then embodied in S. 1320).

In addition, the convention resolution committed the NAACP to work toward "the elimination of the segregated principle as it is now entrenched in all arrangements for medical care as applied to Negroes" (U.S. Senate, Committee on Labor and Public Welfare. Subcommittee on Health 1947, 1092). The NAACP was opposed to the "separate-but-equal" type of provision found in Hill–Burton as "the profession of separate, but equal facilities for the care of negro population . . . has always been a myth, and would prove again to be a myth should it be attempted" (U.S. Senate, Committee on Labor and Public Welfare, Subcommittee on Health Legislation 1949, 506). The NAACP was similarly opposed to plans to augment voluntary prepayment plans on the basis that "where these plans have already appeared and are operating, besides being little available to Negroes on an economic basis, they have been closed to them by reason of racial discrimination as well" (U.S. Senate, Committee on Labor and Public Welfare, Subcommittee on Health Legislation 1949, 506).

The NMA, representing the nation's African American physicians, was similarly supportive of national health insurance until mid-1949. Illustrative of the perceived implications of national health insurance for issues of racial discrimination in health services, the AMA president-elect, in attempting to convince the NMA to withdraw its support for national health insurance, argued that "claims that compulsory health insurance would remove discrimination were 'gravely mistaken.'" He argued that "the highest law of the land, the Constitution of the United States, expressly outlaws prejudice on account of race, creed, or color. This in itself proves that legislation is not sufficient to eliminate the blots of bigotry and race prejudice" (NYT 1949e). Considering that the AMA itself was segregated, this was compelling, if highly ironic, logic. The NMA backed away from its earlier endorsement of national health insurance at its annual convention in August 1949, having received assurances that the AMA, in return, would allow the election of African American members to the AMA House of Delegates.[4]

The support of African American organizations for national health insurance had significant consequences for the politics of national health insurance. First, NAACP support of national health insurance reduced the latitude for southern congressional representatives to support it. The NAACP was the focus of prosegregationist opposition to the civil rights program, and few southern congressional representatives willingly risked favoring a proposal also publicly endorsed by the NAACP.

Second, as a result of the increasing reliance of the Democrats on the support of African American voters, the NAACP position limited the administration's latitude to pursue compromises that might been acceptable to the AMA. For example, the NAACP was "unequivocally and unalterably opposed" to any public health insurance or voluntary prepayment proposals that granted any significant control to the AMA:

> More than civic groups, affiliates of the American Medical Association have been resistant to efforts to obtain relaxation of restrictions against Negro physicians and segregated practices against Negro patients. . . . The National Association could not have confidence in the equitable administration of a program which would be controlled by an organization with the record of the AMA in respect to the Negro.[5] (U.S. Senate, Committee on Labor and Public Welfare, Subcommittee on Health 1947, 1094)

In light of Democratic efforts to court the African American vote and the evident antipathy of the NAACP toward the AMA, it is not surprising that the approach taken by nonsouthern congressional Democrats, some senior administration officials, and President Truman himself toward the AMA was, as discussed below, deliberately antagonistic.

Framing Opposition to National Compulsory Health Insurance

Opposition to national health insurance was framed in language that evoked the language of opposition to civil rights. Much has been made of the devastating effect to which symbolic terms of the debate—especially the term "socialized medicine"—were put. However, the tagging of Truman's health plan as socialized medicine by various opponents—especially the AMA—was not a particularly original or ingenious strategy. Most other progressive social legislation at the time wore the same label—the easiest and most common approach to opposing any progressive social legislation.[6] The real question is, what was it about health services, specifically, that made the socialist tag so politically potent?

Substantively, the single most powerful weapon in the arsenal of opponents of national compulsory health insurance was the issue of doctor choice—the freedom of patients to choose their doctors and vice versa. While salaried doctors were never part of the proposed plan (a point well understood by the plan's leading opponents), this was portrayed publicly as a central element—if not *the* central element—of the Truman plan even as late as 1951 (*Congressional Record* 1949, 12003–4). Shifting doctors' status from that of private practitioners to that of salaried federal employees was widely taken to mean that doctors would no longer have free choice to refuse to see particular patients and that patients would be limited in their choice of doctor (*Congressional Record* 1949, A1530).

For example, the "most widely noted" pamphlet of the 1949 AMA campaign against national health insurance claimed that the federal government's intention was to "dominate the medical affairs of every citizen—through administrative lines from the central government in Washington—down through State, town, district, and neighborhood bureaus"; that the federal government would "assume control not only of the medical profession, but hospitals—both public and private"; and that "the compulsory system inevitably means . . . doctors are assigned to patients and patients to doctors" (Poen 1979, 145–50). Proponents of compulsory health insurance repeatedly reiterated that patients' and doctors' freedom of choice would be, under all proposed legislation, explicitly protected (*Congressional Record* 1945, 10790–91, 10820; *Congressional Record* 1949, A236–7, A1534–5). Despite this, senior AMA officials and other opponents of national health insurance continued to claim that doctors would not be able to choose their patients (*Congressional Record* 1949, A1407).

To the degree that national health insurance was thought to entail doctors becoming federal employees, it posed a direct challenge to segregation in health and physician services. For example, the petition to Congress presented by the state legislature of Mississippi against the Truman health plan does not even mention health insurance. Rather, it memorializes Congress "not to federalize the practice of medicine" or to "enact any proposed legislation, the effect of which is to bring the practice of medicine in this country under direct Federal direction and control" (*Congressional Record* 1950, 5673). Of course, as the proposed national health insurance plan could in no way have been construed to entail the federalization of the medical profession, such statements were obviously calculated to have maximum political impact. In Mississippi in this period the "federalization of medicine" clearly implied a direct challenge to segregationist practices.

Moreover, by framing opposition in the language of choice, opponents reflected and evoked the language of "choice" that was so central to opposition to civil rights in the South. Fair employment practices legislation as well as antisegregation legislation were argued to pose a threat to the civil rights of white southerners by limiting their ability to "choose" their employees as well as to "choose" with whom they would associate (*Congressional Record* 1948, A1864, A2338, A4797). Restricting the right to "choose" patients or doctors could similarly be seen to challenge segregation in health services. It is certainly revealing that, in later debates over medical insurance in Canada, compulsory programs were also widely labeled as socialistic, and doctors vigorously demanded "choice." In these debates, however, choice referred almost exclusively to the manner in which doctors would be compensated. The issue of doctor choice of patient and vice versa never emerged as a significant issue in these debates—remaining an issue peculiar to American health insurance debates.

Public Opinion on National Compulsory Health Insurance

Public support for national health insurance declined considerably from the mid-1940s to the late 1940s. While it is difficult to fully plumb the reasons for this decline given the available data, circumstantial evidence suggests significant effects arising from the link between national health insurance and civil rights—especially in the South.[7]

Public opinion data clearly indicate that racial integration of medical services was a divisive issue among Americans in the mid-1940s—not only in the South. In 1946 fully 50 percent of a national sample responded that they would not like it if they had a Negro nurse.[8] These data suggest the magnitude of resistance that would be generated by proposals raising the specter of the racial integration of medical services. The level of concern over racial integration of health services and the degree to which this concern would receive official sanction in the South is further evident in the implementation, around the same time, of various state laws requiring the segregation of the blood supply.

Shifts in public support for national health insurance in the South are suggestive of the developing link between national health insurance and the issue of civil rights over the mid to late 1940s. In 1945 residents of the South were, across all size-of-place categories, more supportive of compulsory national health insurance (provided under the auspices of Social Security) than the national average (see table 3.1). This pattern challenges the conventional wisdom that public opinion in the

Table 3.1   Support for National Health Insurance (Social Security), United States, by Region, 1945

Question: Do you think it would be a good idea . . . if the Social Security law also provided for paying for the doctor and hospital care that people might need in the future? (% supporting)

	All Regions %	The South %
Total	64	66
+ 500,000	70	—
100,000–499,999	59	64
10,000–99,999	68	72
2,500–9,999	64	65
Under 2,500	59	63
Farm	59	68

Source: Schiltz 1970, 138.

South was more resistant to state intervention per se than in the rest of the country. At the same time, it is crucial to recognize that proposals to extend health insurance through Social Security would likely have received greater public support in the South than more comprehensive national health insurance schemes. As outlined above, Social Security, the contributory pension component of the New Deal, had been made acceptable to the southern congressional representatives only by explicitly excluding agricultural workers and domestic servants—a compromise that helped avoid any challenge from the program to the racial status quo in the South (Quadagno 1988). Extending health insurance through Social Security implied directly replicating this compromise.

In 1949 public opinion in the South was significantly less supportive of the Truman plan for national health insurance (22 percent support) than was the case across the nation more broadly (33 percent support)(see table 3.2.). This is surprising considering that only four years earlier public opinion in the South had been more supportive of federal health insurance than national public opinion. To the degree that health insurance was increasingly perceived as being linked to racial integration, these patterns of regional variation in support for national health insurance are not surprising. Support for Truman's civil rights program also received, by far, the lowest levels of public support in the South, and in 1949 opposition to Truman's civil rights program was four times higher in the South than, for example, in New England (see table 3.3).

Conventional Interpretations of the Failure of National Compulsory Health Insurance, 1945–52

Existing interpretations of the failure of national health insurance in this period tend to focus on the role of the AMA in blocking reform or, alternatively, on the role of expanding voluntary insurance coverage in limiting the political prospects of public health insurance—with such explanations situating both these factors

Table 3.2   Support for National Health Insurance, Various Options, United States, by Region, 1949 (Percentage)

Question: Which of these two plans [for health insurance] would you, yourself, prefer . . .

	Truman Plan	AMA Plan	Neither	No Opinion
TOTAL	33	47	7	13
New England/Mid-Atlantic	38	40	7	15
Far West	37	47	5	11
East Central	31	52	6	11
West Central	27	52	4	17
South	*22*	*52*	*11*	*15*

Source: Strunk 1949, 358.

Question: Which of these two plans [for health insurance] would you, yourself, prefer . . . : the proposed plan of the Truman administration which would require a deduction like Social Security from all salary checks (or wage envelopes) and which would provide all employed persons and their families with insurance for medical, dental, and hospital expenses; or the proposed plan of the American Medical Association which would encourage more people to take out medical and hospital insurance with organizations like the Blue Cross or private insurance companies, with the Government providing money to states and local communities to take of poor and unemployed people who can't afford proper medical attention? [Each respondent was handed a card describing the two plans.]

within the framework of highly fragmented political institutions. Undoubtedly both were important factors shaping developments in this period. However, analyses that attribute too much significance to the AMA's role or the political constraints posed by voluntary private insurance (examined more fully below) risk understating the importance of other dynamics—especially those generated by the politics of race.

The Role of the AMA

Numerous analyses of health insurance in the United States have stressed the over-whelming power of the AMA (Starr 1982, 279, 369; Morone 1990, 255–6; Skocpol 1996, 536–9; Quadagno 2005, esp. 17–47). Much has been made of the AMA's organizational power and financial resources as well as the ostensibly devastating effect of its propaganda efforts—especially its massive 1949 campaign against the

Table 3.3   Support for Civil Rights Program, United States, by Region, 1949 (percentage)

Question: How do you feel about Truman's civil rights program? Do you think Congress should or should not pass the program as a whole?

	Pass	Not Pass	No Opinion	Unfamiliar with Program
New England and Mid-Atlantic	32	14	14	40
East Central	31	18	16	35
Far West	26	20	14	40
West Central	23	19	19	39
South	*13*	*58*	*10*	*19*

Source: Strunk 1949, 156.

Truman plan. Contrary assessments of the AMA's role, however, have concluded that its power was largely illusory (see Harris 1966, 26 passim; Marmor 1970, 114 passim). While the AMA undoubtedly played a highly visible role in the campaign against national health insurance, a number of factors suggest that it was not as powerful as has often been portrayed.

For the most part the AMA's tactics and propaganda efforts were often clumsy. As a result, the AMA's publicity campaigns "had drawn a good deal of criticism from the public at large because of the outlay of money involved, which was enormous, and the tactics employed, which were often questionable" (Harris 1966, 35). While the labeling of national health insurance as "socialistic" was certainly not original, the AMA took this portrayal of national health insurance to sometimes surprising lengths. This extremism was embodied most vividly in the AMA-fabricated claim that it was a central tenet of socialist philosophy that health insurance was the "keystone to the arch of the socialist state." The AMA's strategy was publicly derided, even by opponents of national health insurance, as "not being intelligent": "It has ranted against socialization as though the mere word had conjuring powers" (Thompson 1948). The purple rhetoric of the anti-health-insurance campaign was pushed even further by the National Physicians Committee (NPC), which, while not officially linked to the AMA, had been repeatedly endorsed by the AMA. (The NPC ultimately was disbanded as a result of its track record of embarrassing public relations fiascos, including charges of racism and anti-Semitism [NYT 1948, 1949j.])

The AMA was also beset by internal challenges at both the leadership and membership levels. Just as the AMA was pushing its campaign against national public health insurance into high gear, divisions in the AMA leadership received widespread media coverage. A dispute between the AMA board of trustees and the most prominent AMA spokesman, Morris Fishbein, the long-time editor of the *Journal of the American Medical Association,* broke into the open at the annual AMA convention in 1949. The board of trustees placed a gag order on Fishbein and, in a "bombshell" announcement, removed Fishbein from his various posts (Haseltine 1949; Laurence 1949b). The latter move threatened "an open breach in the ranks of the AMA" and made front-page news (Laurence 1949a).

Also receiving considerable media coverage was internal dissent at the membership level from splinter groups challenging the AMA leadership over its stand on national health insurance. These groups included the Physicians' Forum but, more important, the County of New York chapter of the AMA and the Michigan state chapter of the AMA (NYT 1949c, 1949d; *Washington Post* 1949a, 1949b; *Detroit Free Press* 1949). The New York chapter ultimately refused to have its members pay the $25 assessment on each AMA member to fund the 1949 publicity campaign against national health insurance—a move that drew attention to rifts within the AMA.

The effect of the AMA campaign on public opinion is unclear. Undoubtedly, opposition to the Truman health plan grew over the period in question while support declined (see figure 3.1). These shifts took place, however, in a broader context, one in which nearly half of all survey respondents had either not heard of the national health insurance proposal or, if they had heard of it, did not have an

Figure 3.1   Public Support for National Health Insurance (Truman Proposals), United States, 1945–50

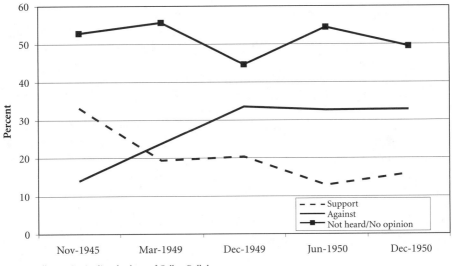

Source: *Gallup Brain*. On-line database of Gallup Poll data.

opinion on the plan—a significantly higher proportion of the population than those who opposed the plan.

When those who had heard of the plan were asked in January 1949 what they thought were the best arguments for or against the plan, more than half either gave no answer or had no opinion—just over a quarter of respondents had heard of the plan and had an opinion about the best arguments in favor and against. Of those who had heard of the plan, only 4.7 percent responded in December 1949 that the best argument against the plan was that it was "socialistic"—down from 5.6 percent in January of 1949 *before* the AMA's massive publicity campaign.[9] These public opinion data fit with the assessment of the AMA's publicity campaign as "no more than a furious bit of shadow-boxing" (Harris 1966, 47).

Nevertheless, the AMA has been widely portrayed as determining the fate of national health insurance. In part, this is due to the visibility of the AMA in these debates. It is also, however, largely the result of a deliberate political strategy of supporters of national health insurance. Unable to get national health legislation through Congress, in no small part because of the recalcitrance of southern Democrats, Truman "responded with vitriolic criticism of the American Medical Association as the public's worst enemy in the effort to redistribute medical care more equitably. . . . Lambasting the AMA was one way of coping with this executive–legislative stalemate" (Marmor 1970, 13).

In keeping with this strategy of focusing blame on the AMA, supporters of national health insurance portrayed the AMA as a small, powerful, and well-funded group that was waging a propaganda war against a program that would benefit average Americans. The 1949 AMA campaign was referred to by one congressional sponsor of national health insurance as "one of the shrewdest, one of the most calculating, and one of the most cold-blooded lobby operations in American history" and by another as "the biggest, most powerful, and most unscrupulous lobby in America" (*Congressional Record* 1949 A3173, 11531). Paradoxically, the latter would go on to taunt the AMA: "The American Medical Association was my chief opponent in the election last fall. I know their methods. I know that they have very little influence at the ballot box; in fact, their opposition got me so many votes that I won last fall by the largest majority I ever received" (*Congressional Record* 1949, 11532).

This criticism of the AMA was highly paradoxical. Administration officials and congressional supporters of national health insurance painted the AMA as a powerful force blocking public health insurance reform while simultaneously adopting a deliberately confrontational posture toward it—presumably a strategy that would have been avoided against a more highly feared adversary. After the 1945 election Roosevelt, according to one of his advisers on the issue of national health, "was clearly looking forward to doing battle with those fellows in Chicago. . . . He seemed amused by their political pretensions" (Harris 1966, 29). Of course, events intervened and it was Harry Truman, along with congressional supporters of national health insurance as well as senior administration officials, who took on the AMA. The AMA was publicly accused of everything from "bad faith and low ethical standards," "blindness and arrogance," to outright lying "in the pattern of other dictators" (*Congressional Record* 1949, A1152, 11531; 1950, A1875). Ewing himself would publicly refer to the entire AMA membership as being composed of "not only fat cats but fraidy cats" whose opposition to any kind of social change, as "frightened men," was driven by fear (*Congressional Record* 1950, A4072).

The AMA's involvement may have been a necessary element in defeating the national health insurance plan, but it was not sufficient. If the AMA's involvement was decisive, it was so because the balance of pro-insurance and opposition forces in Congress—including the critical opposition of southern representatives—allowed it to be. To the extent that the AMA was widely portrayed as all-powerful, this was, to a significant degree, the result of a deliberate strategy of proponents of national health insurance including the Truman administration's strategy to deflect criticism of its own ability to fashion a legislative program with the support of its own southern Democratic caucus. Attacking the AMA held considerable political appeal for northern congressional Democrats as well as the Truman administration—being, among other things, consistent with their strategy to appeal to African American voters.

Voluntary Health Insurance Coverage

Recent interpretations of the failure of national health insurance have focused on the role of voluntary health insurance in limiting the political prospects for public health insurance (Hacker 1998; Gottschalk 2000; Hacker 2002; Béland and Hacker 2004). These works have argued that expanding voluntary insurance coverage reduced popular demand for public coverage as well as created a set of interests, including commercial and not-for-profit insurance providers, hostile to government intervention in the health insurance field. The decline in public support for public health insurance from 1945 to 1949 has thus been attributed to the rise of voluntary insurance coverage "occurring as it did in conjunction with the AMA's postwar public relations blitz" (Hacker 2002, 234). However, this interpretation does not adequately account for the disjuncture between regional patterns in voluntary insurance coverage and regional patterns of support for national health insurance.

Public support for the Truman plan was lowest, by a considerable degree, in the South (see table 3.2). At the same time, coverage by voluntary insurance was also lowest in the South, with only 55 percent of the population having voluntary coverage in 1958 (Somers and Somers 1961, 366). Conversely, public support for the Truman plan was highest in the Northeast, which, in turn, also had the highest rates of voluntary insurance coverage, with fully 75 percent of those in the Northeast having hospital coverage. Had national patterns of public support mirrored those in the Northeast where voluntary insurance coverage was highest, national health insurance might well have passed.

These regional patterns of voluntary insurance coverage and support for public health insurance suggest that support for national health insurance was significantly shaped by factors other than the level of voluntary health insurance coverage. In the South, the low level of support for national health insurance is more compellingly explained by public perceptions of a link between national health insurance and federal antisegregation policies than the displacement effect resulting from voluntary coverage.

The Denouement: Hospital Insurance for the Aged

By 1951 Truman had officially instructed senior administration officials to begin work on a plan for more limited public health insurance coverage. An alternative, based on providing hospital insurance coverage under the rubric of Social Security, had been developing within the FSA since 1949 and was publicly unveiled in early 1952 (Ball 1995, 64). The plan dramatically narrowed the proposed coverage in terms of population and the range of services covered. After 1951 this proposal—which later to became known as Medicare—dominated the strategy of proponents of national health insurance (Marmor 1970, 13).

The issue of which groups would be covered had been as crucial as the question of which health services would be covered. Benefits for the elderly (as opposed to children and pregnant women, for example) were "advocated solely because it seemed to have the best chance politically" (Ball 1995, 62–63). The well-established and politically popular Social Security program provided an attractive basis for providing health insurance benefits. As Robert M. Ball, who was deeply involved in developing the alternative program, noted: "The slogan became 'health insurance through Social Security.' . . . Much was meant by these references to Social Security, some of it explicit and some subliminal" (1995, 65). Most notably, this approach replicated the major compromises on issues of race inherent in the New Deal. Social Security coverage would be extended only to regularly employed farm workers and domestic laborers beginning in 1954—after the "Medicare" approach had come to dominate the strategy of health insurance reformers.

Conclusion

The politics of race were central in ensuring that national health insurance proposals in the Truman era failed. Proposals for national health insurance were inextricably bound up with the politics of civil rights and presented a serious challenge to segregation in the South—a challenge that southern congressional representatives had sufficient power to resist.

Given the political conditions of the period, national health insurance may well still not have passed even if racial politics had not played a significant role in determining this outcome. Conversely, the powerful dynamics generated by the politics of race meant that national health insurance would not likely have passed even if the AMA had taken a much more moderate approach in its opposition to compulsory health insurance. Similarly, it does not appear that national health insurance would have passed had voluntary private insurance coverage been less widespread.

Finally, the failure of national health insurance cannot be attributed simply to the institutional fragmentation of the American system. Considering the strident opposition to national health insurance within the Democratic Party, the measure would not likely have passed even under a less fragmented legislative system such as a parliamentary system. In such systems, sectional opposition can be powerfully exercised within the governing party's cabinet and caucus as well as through federal systems' state or provincial governments. Had national health insurance in Canada faced sectional resistance of a weight and vigor comparable to that of the southern resistance to health insurance in the United States, it would not have been enacted.

Southern resistance combined with powerful resistance from other quarters resulted in the administration having to develop an alternative proposal that would re-create the racial compromises of the New Deal—offering health insurance through Social Security, which excluded large portions of the African American population in the South. This approach became embedded and, even as the constraints to a federal program posed by the politics of race began to ease, shaped the federal approach to the next round of reform.

CHAPTER FOUR

The Medicare Package, 1957–65

> We marvel not simply at the passage of this bill, but what we marvel at is that it took so many years to pass it.
>
> President Lyndon B. Johnson

> Medicare did not by accident follow by less than eleven months the passage of the Civil Rights Act.
>
> David Barton Smith, *Health Care Divided*

A S HAD BEEN THE CASE during the Truman reforms, the politics of public health insurance reform remained entangled with the politics of civil rights through the Medicare era. As David Barton Smith argues,

> Other than the general ebb and flow of electoral politics, the struggle for national health insurance has been described essentially as a self-contained process of vested interests and advocates. In reality, the boundaries between the civil rights struggle during this period and the battle that led to the passage of Medicare were far more blurred in the minds of both protagonists and the public at large. . . . The civil rights legislation and the Medicare and Medicaid legislation shared much more than just a point in time and a combined set of political events that provide an opportunity for action. The cast of characters in both overlapped. (1999, 115–16)

When legislation for public hospital insurance for the elderly was introduced in 1957, it had little chance of passing—yet, by 1965 it had become law.[1] This outcome is largely the result of shifts in the dynamics generated by the politics of race resulting from critical developments such as the passage of the Civil Rights Act. Just as changing conditions allowed for passage of the Medicare/Medicaid package, the intertwining of public health insurance and civil rights had important implications for the specific design of these programs. The resulting structure of the package of programs, their design characteristics, and the delay in the passage of the Medicare legislation, in turn, had important implications for the path of health care reform, helping to explain why expansions of public health insurance were not forthcoming.

Lower case "medicare" is used throughout to refer to the general proposal for a program of hospital insurance for the elderly. "Medicare" is used to refer to the program of public insurance for hospital care (Part A) and medical care (Part B) as actually passed under the Medicare legislation. "Medicare package" refers to Medicare (Parts A and B) as well as Medicaid (medical insurance for low-income persons), which was also passed under the Medicare legislation.

The Politics of Medicare

Medicare was introduced in Congress in 1957 with apparently little chance of passing. Eight years later an expanded version of the proposal, embodied in the Medicare Act, finally passed. It provided for contributory hospital care insurance and premium-based insurance coverage for physician care for eligible Social Security beneficiaries as well as federal grants-in-aid to the states for health insurance for people with low income. Standard accounts of the genesis of Medicare typically attribute the delay in its passage to resistance from the AMA and fiscal conservatives in Congress including Republicans and southern Democrats. Conventional wisdom argues that the Democratic landslide in the 1964 election gave the Johnson administration the political capital to overcome these obstacles. Once it appeared certain that Medicare legislation would pass, the dynamics surrounding its legislative passage were expansionary, and the final package that emerged was broader than any proposals considered to that point. It has often been argued that this expansionary dynamic was the result of a deliberate attempt to forestall the further expansion of public health insurance by "building a fence" around Medicare. The final Medicare package is also often attributed, in retrospect, with having built that fence by providing categorical public health insurance to those least likely to be adequately served by private, voluntary insurance. In contrast with this conventional account, the following sections argue that developments in the politics of race and civil rights were a key element in explaining the shifting political fortunes of medicare over this period.

The Failure to Pass Legislation, 1957–64

When proposals for public hospital insurance coverage for the aged through Social Security reemerged on the political agenda in the late 1950s, the program promised to pose a major challenge to segregated health services if passed. First, Social Security coverage had been extended to agricultural workers and domestic servants in the mid-1950s. In contrast to when it was first conceived in the late 1940s, extending coverage for hospital care through Social Security would, by 1957, include—rather than exclude—most southern African Americans.

Second, the *Brown* decision of 1954 had constitutionally struck down the separate-but-equal doctrine. Federal legislation that was based on the principle of separate-but-equal—such as the Hill–Burton program for hospital construction—seemed likely to be successfully challenged. At the same time, however, the reach of the Hill–Burton law was relatively limited and, even if its separate-but-equal clause were to be struck down, the impact on the segregated health services system would be similarly limited. Any new federal legislation could certainly not include a separate-but-equal clause as had Hill–Burton. Thus, if there were no *new* federal programs for health insurance, there would be no mechanism by which hospital desegregation could be forced on southern states.

Finally, by 1957, it was increasingly clear that civil rights organizations would put as much pressure as possible on the government to ensure that new federal programs enforced desegregation. African American organizations, which had largely been focused on racial segregation in education, were beginning to publicly turn their efforts to challenging segregation in health services. The most visible of these efforts were the annual Imhotep Conferences sponsored by the NAACP, NMA, and National Urban League, the first of which was held in 1957 (NAACP 1957a, 219). The Imhotep conference grew in public visibility—by 1962 receiving a greeting from President John F. Kennedy acknowledging that racial discrimination in hospital practices was an "obvious barrier" to the administration's goals of ensuring that "needed medical care and health services . . . be within the reach of all Americans."[2] In 1957 the NAACP also set, as one its five-year goals, the "free access to non-segregated health services" (1957b, 561).

The threat posed by the medicare proposals to segregated health services ensured that, from the point when Democrat Aimé Forand introduced legislation in 1957, it would be southern congressional representatives who provided the bedrock of opposition to the proposed program. This opposition was channeled through southern control of some of the most powerful committees in Congress. According to Robert Ball, who would become commissioner of Social Security in 1962, the main obstacles to the passage of medicare legislation were Wilbur Mills (D-AR) in the House and Robert Kerr (D-OK) in the Senate. Kerr, the chairman of the Senate Finance Committee, would later be described to have considered defeating medicare to be a "religious mission" (Anderson 1970, 266). For his part, Mills, undoubtedly one of the most influential figures in the congressional process having become chairman of the powerful House Ways and Means Committee in 1957, also strongly opposed the bill.

Popular resistance to desegregation placed considerable pressure on southern congressional representatives. The *Brown v. Board of Education* decision had "crystallized southern resistance to racial change" (Klarman 1994, 82). This backlash against civil rights manifested itself in a strategy of "massive resistance"—the use of whatever means necessary, including violence, to maintain segregation in the South. In a noteworthy coincidence of timing, the first medicare bill was introduced and Mills acceded to the most powerful committee post in the House in the same year that the attempted integration of Central High in Little Rock precipitated a national crisis that ended only with the use of federal troops to enforce the Supreme Court's decision in *Brown*. As one of the many repercussions of the incident, the sitting Democratic congressman representing Little Rock (soon to become part of Mills's congressional district) who had tried to mediate the crisis, was decisively defeated in the following election (Sundquist 1968, 238). In the wake of this defeat, "southern politicians were vying with one another in postures of defiance against the Supreme Court. Southern legislators were competing in the design of legal means to maintain segregation" (Sundquist 1968, 238).

Mills already had established segregationist credentials, having signed the 1956 "Southern Manifesto" in opposition to the *Brown* decision, and he consistently remained opposed to any federal involvement in matters related to race (Zelizer 1998, 133). The shifting position of the Democratic Party on civil rights continued to pose a serious electoral problems for Mills—especially after his district was redrawn to include Little Rock (Zelizer 1998, 133; Marmor 1970, 45). Undoubtedly, medicare "in the minds of many Little Rock voters would be too closely associated with an excessive role for the federal government in social welfare policy" (Marmor 1970, 49).

Debates over an alternative health insurance proposal sponsored by Kerr and Mills highlighted the fact that the main issue in the public health insurance debates was not disagreement between fiscal conservatives and liberals, as often portrayed. Kerr and Mills's alternative to medicare, passed in August 1960, provided federal cost-sharing for state provision of medical care to the needy aged.[3] Relative to the medicare proposals, the Kerr–Mills Act was designed to both limit the scope of public health insurance coverage and keep its administration firmly in state hands. However, two elements of the debates surrounding the Kerr–Mills's versus Medicare debates suggest that the central issue was not simply one of disagreement between liberals and fiscal conservatives.

First, as Alvin David, an administration official, pointed out, the difference between northern and southern Democrats "was much sharper on Medicare than it was on any other issue. On any simple liberal versus conservative issue, this cleavage was never this sharp" (1966). Second, the positions of the antagonists were paradoxical: Medicare proponents were "focusing on *all* social security beneficiaries among the aged, proposing *limited* hospital–surgical insurance for them, to be paid for by *regressive* social security taxes; the more conservative welfare advocates proposing *broader* benefits for a small class among the aged—the destitute—and . . . *progressive* federal tax revenues" (Marmor 1970, 37). Third, Kerr–Mills "did far greater violence to some of the basic principles" of the AMA: "The Kerr–Mills bill was a great deal closer to socialized medicine than the [medicare] bill. The new law left the structure and machinery of government medical care entirely up to politicians. To be sure, they were state and local politicians, who had always proved to be more respectful to organized medicine than national politicians" (Harris 1966, 114). Leaving the structure and machinery of public medical care to state and local politicians was critical in forestalling federal interference with the racial status quo.

The passage of Kerr–Mills did not remove medicare from the political agenda. John F. Kennedy, immediately upon election in November 1960, appointed a Task Force on Health and Social Security for the American People to help establish the priorities of the new administration in these areas. The task force, which issued a report two months later, recommended the extension of hospital insurance under the auspices of Social Security. A month later President Kennedy delivered a health message devoted exclusively to the need for such a program. The related legislation, known as the King–Anderson bill, after its congressional sponsors Representative Cecil King (D-CA) and Senator Clinton Anderson (D-AZ), was introduced immediately after the president's message. The bill was, of course, immediately referred to the House Committee on Ways and Means where it disappeared under the opposition of Mills, other southern committee members, and their Republican counterparts. Administration plans for hospital insurance for the aged introduced with slight revisions in 1962 and 1963 met the same fate—in the former case being defeated in the Senate by 31 Republicans and 21 southern Democrats (S. David 1985, 82).

The short-term political strategy of the administration in regards to its inability to overcome the obstacles presented by the southern Democratic contingent was again to "create an image of a powerful AMA to call attention away from its own incapacity to make Congress (and especially the Ways and Means Committee) do its bidding" (Marmor 1970, 114). When the Forand bill was introduced, the AMA immediately announced a major campaign against the proposal, recalling the fight against national health insurance a decade earlier (NYT 1957). The AMA offered itself as a ready target for this administration strategy of blame-avoidance: "Even before the King–Anderson bill was introduced . . . representatives of the Kennedy Administration had begun castigating the AMA. . . . Although clearly the most immediate threat to enactment was the bottleneck within the Ways and Means Committee, it was the AMA and its supporters who drew most of the Administration's fire" (Marmor 1970, 49).

For its part, the AMA used many of the same tactics as it had in the campaign against national compulsory health insurance a decade earlier, including the portrayal of medicare as a threat to freedom of choice for doctors and patients (Starr 1982, 368). The AMA's tactics proved counterproductive, and the effects of its foray into the 1962 election were not impressive.[4] Nevertheless, ignoring numerous earlier editorials that attributed the delay to Mills,[5] the *New York Times* editorialized on the eve of the signing of Medicare that "only the obstinacy of the American Medical Association has stood in the way until now of doing what should have been done decades ago" (NYT 1965a). The latter claim presaged the conventional wisdom, which held sway for at least the next forty years regarding the AMA's role in the medicare saga.

Shifting blame to the AMA helped proponents of medicare reform to put increasing pressure on non-southern congressional representatives. Medicare supporters "could do little to bring direct pressure on the pivotal congressmen in Ways and Means" (Marmor 1970, 50). In part this was because long electoral tenure bestowed relative political insulation on these congressmen. In part, many southern representatives opposed medicare as a federal intrusion into a matter of states rights—a position that did not expose them to electoral vulnerability. Congressional representatives outside the South, however, appeared more vulnerable. Proponents of medicare portrayed "the AMA as an unscrupulous and inordinately powerful interest which was successfully thwarting the public [which] would cause congressional critics of Medicare to suffer guilt by association" (Marmor 1970, 50).

The Passage of Medicare, 1964–65

Various factors contributed to eventually breaking this legislative stalemate, with developments relating to civil rights playing a key role. The most important was the passage of the Civil Rights Act, which had profound implications for federal programs in all policy areas, including public health insurance. The dynamics generated by these developments also had important implications for the final legislative form the Medicare package ultimately adopted.

The Shifting Political Context of Civil Rights

Three important developments, external to the issue of public health insurance per se, changed the context in which health insurance was being debated. The first was a court ruling in *Simkins v. Moses H. Cone Memorial Hospital* that found the separate-but-equal provision of the Hill–Burton law unconstitutional. The second was the passage of the Civil Rights Act. The third was the increasingly evident failure of the southern campaign of massive resistance to forestall integration in public education. As a result of these developments, the end of segregation in health services appeared increasingly inevitable. This shift contributed to tipping the balance in favor of Medicare's passage.

The *Brown* decision had clearly established that the doctrine of separate-but-equal was unconstitutional. In the early 1960s resolutions were introduced in both the Senate (Javits, R-NY) and House (Green, D-OR; Dingell, D-MI) that would have prohibited hospitals employing discriminatory practices from receiving federal Hill–Burton funds (*Congressional Record* 1962, 1044, 1616; JNMA 1962a, 388; JNMA 1962b, 628). These efforts were unsuccessful. Similarly, direct complaints to DHEW by civil rights groups yielded little in the way of concrete results. For example, when confronted with specific complaints regarding discrimination in a North Carolina hospital using Hill–Burton funds, DHEW responded that "since the Act was passed in 1946 no complaint under this provision had ever been brought before the Department and the Department did not know what action it could take were such a complaint to be brought" (JNMA 1962c, 255). In the absence of voluntary federal action—either administrative or legislative—to address the issue of discrimination under Hill–Burton, civil rights activists turned to the courts.

Successful legal action ultimately came with the Supreme Court decision to uphold a lower court's ruling in the case of *Simkins v. Cone*. The case was "the Brown case for hospitals" (Reynolds 1997). Because of the nature of the separate-but-equal exclusion, the Hill–Burton provision requiring nondiscrimination had traditionally been interpreted as relating only to patients and their access to "essential" services and not to segregation of patients within a hospital or discriminatory practices in granting staff privileges.[6] When the Fourth Circuit Court of Appeals struck down the separate-but-equal exemption, leaving only the nondiscrimination clause, the federal government signaled that it would adopt an expansive interpretation of nondiscrimination: "Technically, then any hospital . . . which was built with the use of Hill–Burton funds and which engages in *any* kind of discriminatory practices in regard to admissions, room assignments, staff privileges, etc., now could be considered to be in violation of the law."[7]

After the Supreme Court declined to issue a writ of certiorari, hospitals applying for Hill–Burton funds were required to ensure that no patient would be denied admission on the basis of race, that no professionally qualified person would be denied staff privileges on the basis of race, and finally, that patients would not be segregated within the hospital (Terry 1965, 35; Reynolds 1997). There still was no mechanism to enforce integration on the segregated hospital system more broadly; the Hill–Burton program provided scant leverage over hospitals that had not received Hill–Burton funds or those that did not intend to reapply for Hill–Burton funds (Reynolds 1997). The outcome of this challenge to Hill–Burton, however, signaled that civil rights groups would aggressively use the courts to challenge health services segregation, that the courts would rule against separate-but-equal provision of health services, and that the federal government would aggressively interpret and implement these rulings.

The Civil Rights Act in 1964 went even further. The act had broader implications for segregated health services than the Hill–Burton decision and "brought many more hospitals under the requirements of civil rights legislation because it affected every health program that was funded by the federal government" (Reynolds 1997). Title VI of the Civil Rights Act of 1964 "required non-discrimination in any federally aided program."[8] The Civil Rights Act opened up the possibility for civil rights groups to directly challenge segregated health services through the courts (Reynolds 1997). Crucial to its passage, the civil rights bill—unlike the medicare proposals—did not fall under the purview of Ways and Means or the Senate Finance committee—proceeding instead through the House and Senate Judiciary committees.

Given the Civil Rights Act and the Democratic victory of 1964, which provided an electoral ratification of the administration's aggressive stance on civil rights, it was increasingly clear that resistance to desegregation was no longer an effective long-term political strategy. Federal officials believed that southern representatives would come to see continuing resistance to federal aid, in areas such as health and education, as futile. As southern legislators could no longer hope for federal grant-in-aid programs allowing segregationist practices, federal officials argued that it was better for southern states to get federal grants where they did in fact qualify (Berkowitz 1995, 203).

These developments contributed to a fundamental shift that made the passage of the Medicare legislation possible—easing the resistance of southern lawmakers.[9] Southern representatives were in a paradoxical position in regard to federal programs (Lieberman 1998, 37). Such programs represented injections of federal financial support into a region where it was often desperately needed. On the other hand, federal programs presented the risk of federal intrusion into matters of states' rights—especially the ability to maintain legal segregation. For example, an editorial in the *Arkansas Democrat,* in defending the "sensible" nature of the racial segregation of hospital patients and warning against further federal intrusion, expressed the clear implications of the Hill–Burton ruling as perceived by segregationists:

"Institutions accepting federal funds are subject to federal control when the government decides to assert authority. No doubt should remain anywhere that laws authorizing federal assistance may be reinterpreted to agree with social and political currents which the public didn't foresee at the time the legislation was enacted" (1964).

If the balance between financial reward and risk of federal intrusion tipped too far toward the latter, proposed programs were unlikely to gain sufficient support among the southern Democratic contingent—which itself was not monolithic. The increasing inevitability of desegregation of health services altered the calculation of this balance. Desegregation of health services (for example, through court challenges) in the absence of a federal program (which would otherwise transfer much-needed federal funds to southern states) would be the worst possible outcome from this point of view.

The looming prospect of hospital integration thus generated the possibility for compromise. For their part, southern lawmakers needed to be able to support health legislation without appearing to be promoting hospital integration while the financial incentives would have to be sufficient to help them sell the program politically. For its part, the administration was trying to get a medicare program passed despite its heavily race-laden implications. Officials in the civil rights arm of DHEW recognized that "the leadership of DHEW regard Medicare, primarily, if not solely, as a health insurance program for the elderly, not as a tool for achieving the racial integration of hospitals" (Reynolds 1997, 1852). Nevertheless, the fact that the desegregation of health services was not central to the immediate goals of proponents of medicare should not obscure the degree to which concerns about desegregation of health services underpinned opposition to the program.

The political latitude of southern lawmakers to support the Medicare package was significantly expanded by the administration's deliberate strategy, since at least 1960, of decoupling the issue of health insurance from the issue of civil rights although it was proceeding on both fronts simultaneously—a significant shift in strategy from the late 1940s. There is little doubt that lawmakers on both sides of the issue were clearly aware of the significance of federal programs—especially those that were federally administered—for the issue of segregation. Senator Harry Byrd, chairman of the Senate Finance Committee, which was considering the Medicare legislation, requested clarification from the secretary of DHEW on whether Title VI of the Civil Rights Act would apply. The unequivocal response was that it would (Smith 1999, 120).

Nevertheless, there was no public discussion of this aspect of medicare in either the House or Senate. As Marmor noted: "Almost no one pressed the issue of racially segregated medical services" (1970, 88). In the words of Robert Ball,

We didn't want it brought up legislatively. It would have been a big barrier to passage in the Senate, particularly, if it had been clear that this [Title VI] was going to be applied. I think everybody knew it, but they didn't want to have to go on record about it. So, it was just one of these colloquies on the floor. It was, at our suggestion, [Senator] Ribicoff [D-CT] and somebody else that pinned down the fact: "Is it going to apply? Yes, sure, it is going to apply." And, that was about all that was said.[10] (NASI 2001, 7)

As Arthur Hess would note, keeping discussion of civil rights off the congressional floor was key to the Democratic strategy on medicare. The administration perceived a sharp difference between integration of schools and integration of hospitals: "Johnson went after the schools, but going after the hospitals was a touchy thing because saying that you mix races in the same bedroom, in the same facility, was a tough one for a lot of southern individuals and hospitals to face" (Hess 1996).

The responsibility for ensuring the passage of the medicare legislation was given to DHEW Assistant Secretary Wilbur Cohen, who was well positioned to facilitate such a strategy:

> As much as he favored civil rights, he also strongly believed in the efficacy of the legislative process and saw his main job as passing education and health insurance legislation that would as a matter of course provide benefits to blacks. He did not want civil rights to envelop and derail those issues. . . . He therefore stuck to his traditional role of accommodating congressional leaders rather than challenging them on the issue of civil rights. He tried to be tactful to the southerners on the issue, never agreeing with their views but always being aware of the political realities. "One thing I've learned from experience," he said in commenting on civil rights issues, "you don't have to say everything that's true" (Berkowitz 1995, 178).

In fact, Cohen came to be viewed by liberals as being too willing to compromise with opponents of medicare.

In keeping with the administration's strategy, African American organizations were conspicuously absent from discussions surrounding medicare in the late 1950s and early 1960s including the proceedings of congressional committees—especially in comparison with their vigorous involvement in the late 1940s. While African American groups such as the NAACP and NMA were supportive of the medicare program, they had grave concerns as to whether medicare would, indeed, address the issue of segregation of health services. In a tightly reasoned letter to Social Security Administration (SSA) Commissioner Ball, John A. Kenney of the NMA stated, "Frankly, I am far from assured that any action is being planned by the Department to guarantee the right of Negro physicians to treat patients in hospitals participating in medicare, or to require participating hospitals to accept eligible Negroes as patients."[11] Kenney was particularly concerned about continual public reassurances given by federal officials that the status quo in patient care would not be disturbed and that medicare would not challenge the current hospital by-laws restricting staff to members of local medical societies—many of which in the South continued to practice segregation.

In response to the ambiguity of the federal commitment on hospital desegregation, African American leaders continued to publicly request that Title VI apply to Medicare and Medicaid even after the Medicare legislation had passed. The NMA claimed that the secretary of DHEW had "'refused to allay fears' that it would approve Medicare funds for segregated hospitals" (NYT 1965e). In what the *New*

York Times characterized as a "strong attack" on DHEW, the NAACP and NMA leaders questioned the sincerity of the DHEW secretary and pointed out that, while he met with "conservative elements of the health profession," he refused to meet with the NMA.

The Outcome—The Medicare/Medicaid Package

Once it was clear that some form of health insurance coverage for seniors was a legislative certainty, the dynamic that emerged was expansionary. At the last minute, Mills proposed a bill amalgamating three different versions of reform that was more comprehensive than any of the preceding proposals. The resulting program has often been described as a three-layer cake. The first, Part A of Medicare, was essentially the Democratic plan for contributory hospital insurance for the aged under Social Security. The second, Part B of Medicare, was essentially a revised version of the Republican counterproposals for government-subsidized voluntary insurance for physician care. The third, Medicaid, was a reprise of the 1950 vendor payments under Old Age Security and, later, the Kerr–Mills bill for state-provided insurance for the elderly needy—albeit expanded to also cover the nonaged poor.

THE STRUCTURE OF THE PACKAGE

The conventional interpretation of this expansionary dynamic is that key congressional decision makers believed that the package had to be broad enough to undercut any future impulse to expand the programs—to "build a fence around Medicare" in the words of Mills (Marmor 1970, 79). Others have attributed this expansion to Mills's concern that a program limited only to hospital care under Social Security as proposed by the Democrats would disappoint the public (Starr 1982, 369). While both dynamics may well have been important contributing factors, the expansionary dynamic also had important effects in reducing the resistance of southern congressional caucus as well as effectively building a fence around the application of Title VI of the Civil Rights Act.

The inclusion of Medicare Part B has been argued to be a strategy on the part of Mills to head off Republican opposition and eliminate physician care insurance as a viable alternative to the Medicare package. At the same time, it was also understood by federal officials that Medicare Part B, providing voluntary insurance coverage for physician care, would not be subject to any civil rights requirement (Ball 1995, 69). The advice provided earlier by the DHEW general counsel echoed the general sentiment in the administration on this matter: "It seems to me clear that we should not try to prevent individual doctors from discriminating in their acceptance of patients."[12] As Smith notes, "Physicians were specifically exempted from compliance with Title VI. DHEW chose to avoid a more difficult battle with organized medicine and concluded that Part B of Medicare, which paid for physician services through a voluntary, federally subsidized plan, was a 'contract of insurance' with its subscribers and not a direct grant of public funds" (2005, 7; 1999, 162–63). From a segregationist viewpoint, striking such a compromise at this point would be

much easier than resisting nondiscrimination requirements in subsequent legislation for physician care if it were introduced sequentially after a nondiscrimination
provision had been applied in regard to Medicare Part A.

Expanding the package to include Medicaid achieved two important functions
central to making the program acceptable to southern congressional representatives.
The addition of Medicaid sweetened the deal financially for southern representatives—further tilting the balance between the risk of federal intrusion and the flow
of federal funds toward the latter. Mills had made an earlier offer to administration
officials to trade his support for health insurance in return for a welfare reform bill
being considered by the administration. Mills told federal officials that "he would
tell his constituents that the health insurance provisions were the price of getting
the welfare amendments that would bring tangible benefits to Arkansas" (Berkowitz
1995, 171). Although the welfare bill did not materialize, the inclusion of Medicaid
in the health insurance reform package represented the same kind of trade-off. Not
surprisingly, the matching formula favored poorer states—including all southern
states (Stevens and Stevens 1974, 30). Furthermore, Medicaid was open ended and
did not impose limits either on individual payments for physician services or on
total state expenditures (Stevens and Stevens 1974, 29). Thus, not only did Medicaid
provide further inducements to southern representatives, it did so while posing no
threat to health care providers: "It covered what would otherwise have been bad
debts for hospitals and raised no challenge to private interests in the medical sector"
(Starr 1982, 371).[13]

In doing so, Medicaid also reflected the same compromise implicit in the social
assistance component of the New Deal with regard to respecting states' rights.
Under the ADC program, federal cost-sharing was provided for payments to families with dependent children but eligibility, benefit levels, and administration were
left to the states (Lieberman 1998, 48–56). This compromise had allowed for the
federal government to provide support for aid without challenging states' rights—
relieving southern concerns that cash payments to needy families in the South could
serve to undermine the racial status quo. As a result of state administration, African
American families were, in a number of states, effectively discriminated against in
terms of eligibility as well as average benefit levels (Lieberman 1998, 126–30). In
its reliance on state administration, Medicaid re-created this compromise. Most
important, the Medicaid compromise left enforcement of civil rights provisions to
the states (Wing and Rose 1980, 264). This had been the case under the Kerr–Mills
Act in the year between the passage of the Civil Rights Act and the Medicaid title
when Title VI could presumably have been enforced on health facilities receiving
aid under Kerr–Mills but was not (Wing and Rose 1980, 246).

Crucially, Medicaid created a programmatic space to lodge nursing home care,
which "couldn't very well be left out of a program extending Kerr–Mills" (Vladeck
1980, 51).[14] Including nursing home care in Medicaid helped ensure that this element of health services was not subject to the full application of nondiscrimination
requirements of the Civil Rights Act that federal officials foresaw for hospitals under
Medicare. It had been clear from the outset that a "combination of political events

and the distinctive characteristics of nursing homes themselves had left them insulated . . . from federal efforts to enforce Title VI" (Smith 1999, 237). While the federal government clearly was not willing to countenance segregation in extended-care facilities that would provide residential but also significant levels of medical service to elderly recipients, policymakers certainly had not anticipated integrating small, private nursing homes that primarily provided residential services—especially those that were proprietor occupied. As Smith notes,

> Many saw [Title VI] enforcement in nursing homes as straying across a fuzzy boundary between the public and the intimate private lives of citizens. . . . Many nursing homes were owner-operated converted houses . . . begun in the 1930s by nurses or poor widows. . . . Surely the bill would not force such poor women, trying to eke out a meager existence, to have black men live in their homes? No one, including Kennedy and Johnson, was willing to go that far. . . . Was the federal government going to force race-blind room assignments? Johnson was apparently troubled by that question and saw a clear distinction between the standards that should be imposed on medical facilities and the homes in which people lived. (1999, 160)

This conundrum was resolved by the legislative division of nursing home care into two separate categories—extended care, which would be included in Medicare, and unskilled nursing home care, which would be provided under Medicaid. The former would cover sixty days of post-hospital extended care (requiring 24/7 nursing services and employing at least one registered nurse on a full-time basis) that must be provided in a facility that was either formally affiliated with or had a patient-transfer agreement with a general hospital (Vladeck 1980, 49, 55). Such care, to be eligible for reimbursement under Medicare, would require certification by DHEW, including certification of Title VI compliance. All other nursing home care—which would prove to be the bulk of all nursing home care—would be provided under the auspice of state medical assistance programs (to those who did not exceed maximum financial requirements) and funded through Medicaid with Title VI certification being left to the individual states. As argued below, the inclusion of the bulk of funding for nursing home care in Medicaid would have other critical repercussions on the development of the Medicaid program.

DESIGN CHARACTERISTICS

The specific characteristics of these programs as they were to emerge reflected a key concern of Medicare policymakers—the successful enforcement of civil rights compliance. Addressing the issue of hospital segregation and Title VI compliance was the central challenge in implementing Medicare and an issue with which President Johnson himself became personally concerned—including involvement in discussing plans to use Armed Forces helicopters to airlift patients from noncompliant hospitals in the event that these hospitals were shut down.[15] Effective enforcement of Title VI required a smooth takeoff for the program in all other respects. If Medicare were to falter for any other reason, such as a general doctors' boycott or resistance from hospitals more generally, political pressure would be taken off the hospitals that were resisting Title VI compliance.

This created the context for a package that was extremely favorable to hospitals and the medical profession. First, the programs made provision for fiscal intermediaries (which tended to be Blue Cross and Blue Shield organizations) that would undertake auditing and provide reimbursements to providers from federal funds. This was one of the major compromises worked out by federal officials and southern congressional leaders to assuage the concerns of southern Democrats regarding federal control (Berkowitz 1995, 172, 215). As a result of this provision for intermediaries, which was designed primarily to protect against excessive federal control, "the federal government surrendered direct control of the program and its costs" (Starr 1982, 375). Second, the rules regarding payment to hospitals were extremely favorable to the hospital industry, including, for example, depreciation and capital costs (Starr 1982, 375). Finally, physician services would be reimbursed under Medicare at "customary and reasonable" rates rather than according to a set fee schedule.[16] All three provisions would contribute to the overall escalation of the programs' costs.

The AMA leadership clearly was satisfied with the terms of the deal. Even before the legislation passed into law, the AMA leadership made front-page national news by cautioning members against opposing the pending legislation (NYT 1965b). Among various quarters of the AMA membership, there was pressure for a boycott of the Medicare program even though there was no effective way for doctors to do so.[17] While reluctant to mandate that its members participate in Medicare, the AMA argued strongly against boycotting the program, claiming that doing so would make the organization liable to antitrust prosecution (NYT 1965d). The AMA leadership vigorously defended its position against a boycott at the annual convention of its House of Delegates. This occurred just weeks prior to the passage of the final law—a time presumably when the political impact of such a threat was at its maximum.[18] Coincidentally, the same meeting of the AMA House of Delegates rejected a resolution that "would permit Negro doctors who were barred from local medical societies to obtain direct membership in the AMA"—ratifying a policy that gave segregated local medical societies the ability to deny African Americans hospital staff privileges as well as access to the national organization (NYT 1965c).

The possibility of problems with civil rights compliance created serious constraints on the administration's latitude to enforce tougher terms on the hospital industry and medical profession. As Starr argues, "an administration more concerned with the budgetary consequences of concessions than with smooth take-off would not have yielded as much" (1982, 378). Federal efforts to revise the compromises of 1965 and implement some measure of cost control did not emerge until the early 1970s as Medicare's achievements in terms of civil rights were consolidated.

Implementation—Racial Integration of Health Services

The smoothness of Medicare's takeoff in all other respects allowed top DHEW officials to devote their energies in the first weeks of the program almost singularly to the issue of certifying southern hospitals for Title VI compliance (Marmor 1970, 88). Despite the fact that the Medicare legislation made no mention of segregation of health services or the application of Title VI of the Civil Rights Act, the program would directly challenge segregated hospital care—as legislators on both sides of the issue had been well aware. Wilbur Cohen's recollection (1986, 116) twenty years after the enactment of Medicare reveals how central the issue of civil rights enforcement was at the inception of the program:

> On the day before Medicare went into effect, in every hospital in the South, over every drinking fountain, over every bathroom, over every cafeteria, there were signs reading "White" and "Colored" for separate but presumably equal facilities. On the day that Medicare went into effect in the South, all those signs and separate facilities began to come down. This I think was a singular achievement of Medicare. In one day Medicare and Medicaid broke the back of segregated health services."[19]

Six days after the Medicare program began operating, federal officials publicly declared civil rights compliance a success (Berkowitz 2003, 149). While the extent and immediacy of civil rights compliance is still open to question, there is no doubt that some hospitals receiving Medicare funds allowed segregationist practices well after the program came into effect (see Marmor 1970, 84; Berkowitz 2003, 149). The early claims of federal officials in this regard appear to have been politically motivated—designed to increase pressure on hospitals that were not yet in full compliance with Title VI.

In terms of civil rights enforcement, the approach to nursing home care that had been adopted had a strikingly different impact: "Outside the hospital, the rest of the health care system was never directly affected by the Medicare integration efforts. No effort to inspect nursing homes for compliance was ever mounted" (Smith 2005, 7). For extended-care facilities subject to requirements under Medicare, civil rights enforcement efforts occurred after the hospital certification process had been completed. By the time that HEW's attention turned to certification of extended-care facilities, most of the huge temporary staff that had been put together for hospital certification was no longer available (Wing and Rose 1980, 427). As a result, "Title VI enforcement in nursing homes fell apart before it got started" (Smith 1999, 159). A staff member of the long-term care division of the Office of Equal Health Opportunity later recalled: "We had hoped . . . to follow up on the nursing homes, as we had done with the hospitals. Nevertheless, President Johnson decided during the first part of 1967 that he was not going to require anything. All he was going to do is require a good-faith effort" (Smith 1999, 236). As a result, nursing home certification was based "almost entirely on the assurances and compliance reports, with few site visits" (Wing and Rose 1980, 263).

For nursing homes receiving funding through Medicaid and thus under state compliance authority, the Office of Civil Rights (OCR)—as a separate unit within HEW with the mandate to enforce Title VI—could only monitor state enforcement activities. Wing and Rose note, "This enforcement program has been grossly understaffed and underfunded" (1980, 247). The OCR was fully cognizant of the fact that state compliance efforts were minimal and that many states provided Medicaid certification to nursing home facilities on the basis of paper documentation in the absence of site visits, which had initially been required. At the same time, the OCR itself did not require states to generate or report Title VI compliance-related data. As of 1973, "at least sixteen states had no Title VI certification process at all, and many had no regular monitoring activities" (Wing and Rose 1980, 264).

The lackadaisical application of Title VI to nursing home care is not surprising. The federal position on Title VI enforcement on extended-care facilities through Medicare had always been ambivalent. For unskilled nursing homes ostensibly subject to Title VI requirements through Medicaid, no one would have been surprised—especially given the history of state involvement in battles over desegregation in education—that state-level enforcement was inadequate. This was, however, part of the compromise implicit in the inclusion of nursing home care primarily under the rubric of Medicaid.

Medicare and Medicaid—The Aftermath

Both proponents and opponents of public health insurance expected that the new programs would generate an expansionary dynamic in terms of both population coverage and service coverage (Harris 1966, 64; Marmor 1970, 61; Hacker 2002, 250).[20] Despite public denials, some proponents believed that the Medicare package would be the stepping-stone to universal public health insurance (Berkowitz 2003, 121). Reformers had every reason to be sanguine. They saw the Medicare package as the extension of another earlier means-tested age-limited program—Kerr–Mills—that had failed to head off broader public insurance coverage. Robert Ball captures the logic that motivated reformers: "What history shows us, if you have a category of programs on a means-tested basis, it really helps you get social insurance later on, rather than be a final solution that people point to and say, 'Well, you don't need social insurance because we already have a means tested program.' It doesn't work that way. People are not satisfied with a means-tested program and they will want to reduce the assistance cost by social insurance" (2001). This reasoning, however, overlooked the price that had to be paid in terms of weakened cost control for emphasizing a smooth takeoff in a context of contested civil rights compliance. The surrender of control over costs in the short to medium term placed tight and immediate political limits on program expansion.

Medicare

A central tension in the Medicare program resulted from the initial compromise by which the federal government relinquished control over the fees paid to medical providers and the overall cost of the program (Oberlander 2003, 8). As a result, Medicare soon came to be viewed as financially uncontrollable. Only five years after the inception of the program, a Senate Finance Committee (1970, 1) report flatly stated: "The Medicare and Medicaid programs are in serious financial trouble."[21] The rapidly rising cost of the programs forced reform onto the agenda. The key issue in Medicare reform immediately became one of cost control rather than benefit expansion despite the fact that there were powerful pressures in favor of the latter

(Marmor 2000, 96; Oberlander 2003, 43, 48). Nevertheless, for the next twenty years, benefits remained virtually unchanged. This, in turn, had two effects. First, it exacerbated the tension, which would grow more marked as the costs of medical care increased, between "the promise of Medicare (as understood by the public) to protect the elderly against the potentially devastating costs of medical care and the actual performance of the program in delivering on that promise" (Oberlander 2003, 8) Second, in the absence of program expansion, private supplemental insurance—Medigap policies—came to fill the vacuum and, in turn, contributed to defusing pressures for further program expansion (Oberlander 2003, 49).

As a result of the financial crisis, the evolution of the Medicare program has been marked by a series of reforms designed to control costs. The federal response to the first Medicare bankruptcy crisis in the early 1970s was to create professional standard review organizations in 1972 that were to monitor utilization rates for Medicare services to ensure against misuse or fraud. The reforms were not particularly effective in controlling costs; however, they demonstrated the federal government's concern with cost control and represented a "halting first step" toward asserting federal control over organized medicine in the program (Oberlander 2003, 116–20).

In the 1980s, in response to the second Medicare bankruptcy crisis, the federal government moved to the prospective payment system, which was a system of fixed rates for hospital care (Oberlander 2003). Under this system, adopted in 1983, hospitals were paid on a per-case basis for each patient within a designated diagnostic-related group regardless of the actual cost of treatment. The introduction of the prospective payment system effectively reduced the cost per patient incurred by Medicare relative to private insurance (Oberlander 2003, 125). According to Marmor, this was "the most consequential health initiative of the 1980s" (1994, 23). The need to move away from "reasonable and customary" charges as embodied in the initial Medicare program had become obvious very early in the program's development yet occupied the attention of reformers for nearly two decades before being successfully addressed.

At roughly the same time, Congress attempted to control costs in Medicare Part B by freezing physician fees. Despite a freeze on fees from 1984 to 1986, costs continued to increase because of increases in utilization, creating pressure for tighter regulation and a fixed fee schedule. Part of the rationale was that a fixed fee schedule (based on the "relative value" of the procedure) was expected to favor less expensive primary care over specialized medical care, thus contributing to overall cost control (Oberlander 2003, 128). Congress adopted the fee schedule in 1989 and, at the same time, enacted volume performance standards (a system that would reduce payments in subsequent years for physicians exceeding allowable billing limits) and limits on billing patients for amounts over scheduled rates.

Thus it was a quarter century before the Medicare program got some handle on the issue of cost control—an outcome that political conditions of the mid-1960s had rendered untenable at the program's inception. Even with these reforms, Medicare still represented an open-ended spending commitment for the federal government—a situation that "help set the stage for the political turbulence that hit Medicare in the mid-1990s" (Oberlander 2003, 8).

Medicaid

For its part, Medicaid moved from being a "glittering symbol of the 'Great Society'" to being a political liability by the early 1970s (Stevens and Stevens 1974, xvi). As early as 1966, Medicaid costs were three times the initial DHEW estimates. As a result, "almost as soon as the first program began, a backlash set in" (Stevens and Stevens 1974, 108, 91).

While initial federal restrictions on eligibility for state programs were minimal, reforms in 1967 intended to address cost escalation tied eligibility for Medicaid programs to state-determined AFDC benefits.[22] Debates regarding Medicaid became tied directly to debates regarding cash welfare. By 1972 Medicaid programs could be accurately described as an extension of cash assistance (Stevens and Stevens 1974, 117, 236). As a result of the increasingly welfare-oriented bent of the program, Medicaid began to drop as a political priority.

Despite restrictions on eligibility, costs continued to rise. Large increases in fees were already taking place due to "standardizing-up" as a result of the formalization of doctors' fees based on profiles of usual and customary fees in each area (Stevens and Stevens 1974, 194). As an example, Medicaid costs increased by 57 percent between 1968 and 1970 even though there was only a 19 percent increase in recipients (Stevens and Stevens 1974, 183). Thus in addition to the restrictions on eligibility of 1967, federal restrictions on levels of individual payments to physicians followed in 1970. However, not surprisingly, in cases where physician-dominated organizations such as Blue Shield operated as the fiscal intermediary, states found it difficult to control fees (Stevens and Stevens 1974, 192). Even after a federal fixed fee schedule was implemented, increasing numbers of families eligible for AFDC drove huge growth in program costs. From 1969 to 1973 overall Medicaid costs doubled and were forecast to double again by 1980. By 1970, the consistent response of the states was to "prune back" Medicaid programs (Stevens and Stevens 1974, 261–62).

At the same time, a powerful contrary dynamic had been set in motion by the decision to include nursing home care under the rubric of Medicaid. By 1975 the Medicaid program was already funding the long-term care of more than half of all nursing home residents. As a result, the Medicaid program was transformed from a program providing medical care coverage for the poor to a "key social support for the mainstream elderly" (Grogan and Patashnik 2003a, 836). This shift, as Grogan and Patashnik compellingly argue, has fundamentally shaped the political dynamics of the program as outlined more fully below.

Failure of Comprehensive Reforms

Despite both hopes and fears that Medicare would act as a stepping-stone to expansions of public health insurance, attempts at reform became entangled with ever-increasing fiscal pressures and concerns about spiraling program costs, declining trust in government stemming from Vietnam and Watergate, and increasing pessimism about the ability of government programs to alleviate social problems, including the racial tensions wracking the American political system. Various attempts at public health insurance reform emerged, but none was successful. There were some significant, if limited, reforms that ultimately reinforced the orientation toward private, employer-provided insurance for the working population and public insurance for the aged and poor. However, the basic structure of American public health insurance as it emerged from this period resisted significant change for the next forty years.

Concerns about spiraling health care costs placed broader health insurance reform on the public agenda while simultaneously limiting its chances of success. Proposals for major health insurance reform in this period, including both those for universal public coverage and those for universal coverage based on mixed private and public provision, failed. The broadest proposal for reform was embodied in the Kennedy–Griffiths "Health Security" proposals that would have provided universal, first-dollar insurance for a comprehensive range of medical care— "replacing all public and private health plans in a single, federally operated health insurance system" (Starr 1982, 394). In response President Nixon advocated a plan combining mandated employer-provided insurance with public health insurance for all those not already covered. Under this plan insurance coverage would be universal but not universally public coverage. While there may have been the potential for compromise between the two camps, proponents of universal public health insurance became less disposed to compromise as they became more convinced that Nixon would be forced from office as a result of the Watergate scandal.

While these proposals did not pass, developments in regard to employer-provided health insurance proved significant. The Employee Retirement Income Security Act [ERISA] of 1974 was aimed at ensuring that private pension plans could not be regulated by the states in order to address concerns from large employers and unions regarding inconsistent state regulations as well as state interference with negotiated benefit funds. In doing so, the legislation exempted all benefit programs provided by employers, including health care, from state regulation. Thus, employers who self-insured would be exempt from state laws while the federal legislation did not itself impose federal regulations.[23] Although largely unnoticed at the time, the policy represented a "massive shift in the regulatory environment surrounding health insurance."[24] Hacker (2002, 256, 260) argued that the implications for health insurance reform were also to be profound: "not only had national politicians failed to pass major insurance reforms, but they had also added new hurdles to the already formidable barriers that stood in the way of state leadership."[25]

After this point the prospects for national health insurance reform began to dim as a result, in the first instance, of severe economic recession combined with high inflation. Ironically, while rising costs in the early 1970s made the need for reform "seem all the more urgent; now they made such efforts seem all the more risky" (Starr 1982, 406). This turning point for public health insurance thus coincided with a broader trend: "the end of the postwar growth of social entitlements" (Starr 1982, 405).

Furthermore, public support for government intervention in health care had taken a dramatic reversal following the inception of Medicare and Medicaid. From 1968 to 1976, Coughlin reports (1980, 21) the percentage of respondents of polls choosing the alternative that "government should help people get medical care" dropped from 52 percent to 42 percent. More significantly, the percentage of respondents choosing the alternative that "government should stay out of medical care" increased from 27 percent to 44 percent (see figure 4.1). Thus, by the mid-1970s, for the first time, more respondents felt that government should stay out of health care than were supportive of government intervention.

Illustrative of the racially divided nature of the health insurance issue, African Americans were much more likely than whites to choose the alternative that "government should see that everyone has medical care" and much less likely to choose the alternative that "government should stay out of health care" (Coughlin 1980, 46). The differences between African Americans and whites on this issue were much more significant than differences within either group based on education or income (see table 4.1).

Declining support for government provision of medical care resulted from the financial burdens posed by Medicare and Medicaid, exacerbated by the lessening support for government intervention more broadly. From the early 1970s through the mid-1980s to late 1980s, Great Society programs were increasingly seen to have been an abysmal failure and were charged with having actually exacerbated the problems at which they were aimed.[26] By the late 1970s, even liberal proponents of health insurance reform, including organized labor, had largely abandoned the idea of universal public coverage.[27] In the late 1970s, under the leadership of Senator Ted Kennedy, labor leaders and liberal Democrats proposed a system of universal coverage based on private health plans (that would compete for subscribers) with income-contingent premiums paid to the government (two-thirds of which would

Figure 4.1   Public Attitude toward Government Intervention in Health Care, United States, 1964–76

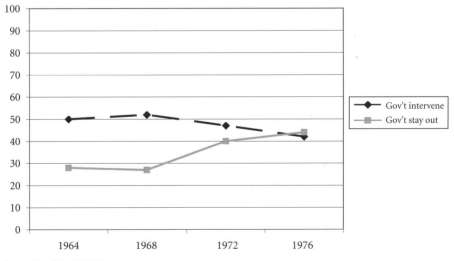

Source: Coughlin, 1980: 21.

Table 4.1 Public Attitudes toward Government Guarantees of Health Care, United States, by Race, 1968 (percentage)

	Did not graduate high school		At least high school diploma		<$8,000 per year		>$8,000 per year		Total sample
	White	Black	White	Black	White	Black	White	Black	
Government ensures everyone has medical care	59	85	41	79	53	84	44	79	51
Government stays out of health care	21	4	35	4	25	3	35	6	27

Source: Coughlin 1980, 46.

be paid by employers) and the government covering the cost for the poor (Starr 1982, 413). For its part, the Carter administration proposed mandated employer-provided insurance, expanded public insurance for seniors and the poor, and set up a public corporation to sell health insurance to those not otherwise covered—although it never aggressively pushed the plan (Starr 1982, 413). Universal public coverage was off the political agenda, and even more moderate proposals such as those of the Carter administration foundered. With the election of Ronald Reagan as president, the issue of national health insurance "vanished like a mirage from American politics" (Starr 1982, 414).

Conclusion

The politics of public health insurance continued to be entangled with the politics of civil rights in the period preceding Medicare's inception. Important external shifts—especially those related to the passage of the 1964 Civil Rights Act—altered the context in which health reform debates took place and opened the possibility for compromise leading to major reform. While southern opposition to federal intrusions in health services was rock solid in 1957, by 1965 southern representatives were willing to accept a federal program so long as they did not have to appear to be supporting the integration of health services. The result was the passage of the Medicare Act in 1965.

The politics of race had three major effects on public health insurance reforms in this period. First, the intertwining of health insurance and civil rights contributed to a significant lag in the passage of the Medicare legislation. This delay pushed further health care reform into a period in which the political conditions were significantly less propitious for expansion of public health insurance. Second, the politics of race also help explain aspects of program structure, such as the inclusion of Medicaid as a trade-off for helping secure southern support for the package as well as the inclusion of long-term nursing home care for the elderly in Medicaid rather than Medicare. Finally, the politics of race and linkage of health insurance reforms to desegregation of hospital care contributed to particular characteristics of the Medicare programs—most notably the lack of cost controls.

The result of the latter was that, virtually from the start, program expansion was not a realistic political possibility, and reform efforts for the following two decades were geared toward cost control. The result of including nursing home care in Medicaid was that the Medicaid program did not become as highly racially identified as other programs such as AFDC and Food Stamps. As a result, debates regarding reform of public health insurance programs in the 1990s did not automatically implicate the issue of race as did other issues, such as welfare reform. This helped generate the opportunity for health insurance reform that the Clinton administration would seize on coming to power.

CHAPTER FIVE

Race and the Clinton Reforms

All of us, we know all about race baiting. They've used that old tool on us for decades. And I want to tell you one thing, I understand this tactic and I will not let them get away with it in 1992.

President William J. Clinton

As CLINTON'S QUOTE so clearly emphasizes, race continued to play a significant role in policy debates in the 1990s. At the same time as health care reform was being debated, a major "culture war" was taking place—reaching its apotheosis in the mid-1990s. Concurrent with making proposals for health reform, Clinton committed to major welfare reform "ending welfare as we know it" and crime control—both issues conjuring up powerfully racialized imagery. While health care reform did not pass, welfare reform took center stage when the Republicans gained control of Congress in 1994. To the Republican congressional majority, welfare reform revolved around the issue of the African American underclass, and conservatives explicitly cast welfare reform as related to the "meltdown" in the black family. At the same time, the 1990s saw the greatest crime war in American history sweeping city streets of young African American men. In the politics of both welfare reform and crime control, race played a powerful role.

Dynamics related to race also powerfully shaped the opportunities for health care reform in the 1990s. They did so, however, in a manner much different than had been the case in the postwar period from 1945 to 1965—remaining latent below the surface of health reform debates. That the relationship between the politics of race and health reform was distinct from earlier periods is not surprising—the major programs of the 1960s had radically shifted the context in which the politics of race and health reform intersected.

Understanding the politics of race in this period is central in understanding how health insurance reform could become one of three central planks of a "New Democrat" presidential contender whose other major platform items—ending welfare and strengthening crime control—were carefully crafted to ensure that he did not end up on the wrong side of the racial divide. As a result of dynamics created by the programs that emerged out of the 1960s, reforming health insurance by the

1990s, including the expansion of coverage to the uninsured, was a political strategy that was highly inoculated against racial backlash. Popular images of the uninsured were not highly racialized in large part because of the perception that the very poor (a category of people that itself has a highly racialized image) already received coverage under existing government programs. At the same time, because of the peculiarities of their historical development, programs such as Medicaid were not perceived primarily in racial terms nor had political leaders tended to cast them in this light. These factors helped generate an opportunity for major reform.

In terms of its failure, dynamics relating to race contributed to an overall context that was inhospitable to health insurance reform. First, the heightened racial charging of the American political system in the early 1990s—a context to which the Clinton administration's proposals for welfare reform and crime control contributed—helped undermine general public support for both expansion of federal programs and increases in taxes necessary to fund them. This greatly constrained the Clinton reformers' latitude in designing their package of health reforms. Second, this heightened racial charging also contributed to lowering the public salience of health care relative to issues that more directly played on racial dynamics, such as welfare reform and crime control, where reforms would ultimately be successful.

The Clinton Reforms—An Overview

Not only did President Clinton combine health reform with welfare reform and crime control, but his health reform proposals themselves reflected his carefully crafted approach of championing the middle class—a central focus of his campaign in the Democratic primaries and later in the 1992 presidential election—thus even further minimizing his exposure to the race-baiting of which he was so keenly aware. In the late 1980s and early 1990s, health care reform fit naturally with this middle-class focus. A number of trends had been emerging since the 1970s that caused health care to become a pressing issue for the middle class: rising premiums for employer-provided health insurance, the increasing visibility of health care costs for working Americans through copayments and deductibles, the shift from community rating to experience rating in private insurance plans, and the movement by private insurers toward managed care (Hacker 1997, 12).

Protecting coverage enjoyed by the insured was central to the Clinton plan—extending coverage to the uninsured was not. Despite the fact that the number of uninsured had been increasing significantly in the 1980s, this issue was not of primary political salience:

> In a political sense . . . the uninsured hardly formed a group at all. They were faceless and quiescent, without common ties or identification, and more than a quarter were children. So the growing number of uninsured could not by itself be expected to spur political leaders to action. Something more was needed to create significant public pressures for national health care reform. As it turned out, that something was the intrusion of rising health care costs into the medical security of the middle class" (Hacker 1997, 15).

In fact expanding coverage for the uninsured in many ways seemed instrumental, if not incidental, to the Clinton plan with Clinton believing that expanding coverage was key to effective cost-control.[1]

The plan the Clinton reformers adopted to advance the goal of protecting middle-class coverage could be characterized as inclusive managed competition—an approach predicated on regulating the market-based provision of health insurance in a way that was intended to achieve cost control and universal (primarily private) coverage.[2] Universal coverage would be largely guaranteed through mandating compulsory employer contributions to employee health coverage on a percentage of premium basis. This coverage would have to conform with a government-guaranteed baseline package that would be comparable to typical coverage provided by America's largest corporations. All employers (except those with more than five thousand people) would be required to purchase privately provided insurance through state-approved "health alliances" that would approve the plans employers could offer as choices to their employees. Employees would be able to choose among packages but would have to bear the full cost of premiums above the least expensive plan offered. As the regional alliances would purchase insurance on behalf of large pools of employers from existing insurance companies and health maintenance organizations, competition would exist but would be managed. These large mandatory regional alliances would serve a twofold purpose: creating large pools to ensure broadly based community rating and promoting cost-control through the aggregation of buying power. The latter was expected to encourage the expansion of managed care under health maintenance organizations (HMOs), preferred provider organizations (PPOs), and similar organizations (Skocpol 1996, 44). Finally, the plan included contingent premium caps that would kick in only if managed competition did not sufficiently dampen cost increases.

It was expected that extending insurance coverage through employer mandates would free up funds from the existing Medicare and Medicaid programs.[3] Thus, the proposal included significant cuts to both Medicaid and Medicare. The saved money would then, in turn, be used to subsidize the purchase of health insurance by the unemployed through the proposed regional alliances. The result was that the bulk of funding to cover the uninsured would come, in effect, from employer-paid premiums (Skocpol 1996, 44, 71). This system of managed competition would also be inclusive—every American citizen would be covered by an employer plan, public plan, or government subsidy. President Clinton stressed that his plan envisioned "a private system."[4] Clinton described his proposed system as "personal choice, private care, private insurance, private management, but a national system to put a lid on costs, to require insurance reforms, to facilitate partnerships between business, government and health care providers." By 1994, Clinton would refer to his health reform plan, in contrast with "government insurance," as "guaranteed private insurance."

The Broader Context—'Racial Charging'
of the American Political System

Clinton's focus on the middle class seemed especially politically adroit in the context of the early 1990s, which had witnessed a marked increase in the racial charging—

the degree to which political and policy debates revolved around issues relating to race—of the American political system. In this period public concern with the degree of attention paid to blacks and other minorities was rising. The average net proportion of respondents to polls feeling that blacks and other minorities received too much attention, a proxy indicator of racial backlash, increased over the 1980s and 1990s, with a sharp upturn after 1992, and peaked in 1994[5] (see figure 5.1). By 1994, for the first time, the proportion who believed that the right amount of attention was being paid to blacks and other minorities dipped below those who felt that it was too much. The latter group represented more than one-third of all respondents—having increased from less than one-fifth of respondents a decade earlier.

By the mid-1990s, the context for expanding federal services or increasing taxes was highly unfavorable, and public perceptions relating to race were clearly significant in reducing support for such expansion. In 1995 more than 54 percent of respondents supported reductions in federal services and taxes, and more than 45 percent of all respondents cited too much spending on low-income minorities as a reason (see figure 5.2). The latter group outstripped all respondents who supported expanding federal services.[6]

Figure 5.1   Perceptions Regarding Attention Paid to Blacks and Other Minorities, United States, 1982–94

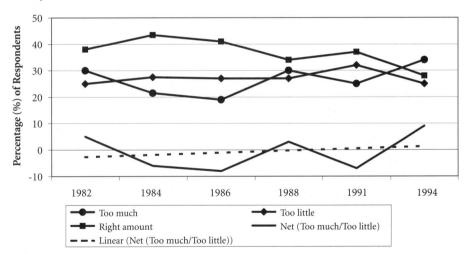

Source:
Los Angeles Times. 1982. No title. 7 January 1982. Accessed from Roper Center for Public Opinion Research online via LexisNexis. [Accession Number: 0079223]
———. 1984. No title. 15 October 1984. Accessed from Roper Center for Public Opinion Research online via LexisNexis. [Accession Number: 0080310]
———. 1986. No title. 9 July 1986. Accessed from Roper Center for Public Opinion Research online via LexisNexis. [Accession Number: 0077082]
———. 1988. No title. 10 July 1988. Accessed from Roper Center for Public Opinion Research online via LexisNexis. [Accession Number: 0077664]
———. 1991. No title. 25 September 1991. Accessed from Roper Center for Public Opinion Research online via LexisNexis. [Accession Number: 0163110]
———. 1994. No title. 31 May 1994. Accessed from Roper Center for Public Opinion Research online via LexisNexis. [Accession Number: 0231067]

Figure 5.2   Support for More/Less Federal Services, United States, 1995

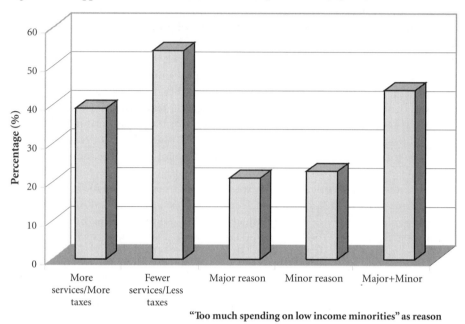

Sources: Harvard University and Kaiser Family Foundation. 1995. *Washington Post/Harvard/Kaiser Family Foundation Race Relations Poll.* 1 December 1995. Accessed from Roper Center for Public Opinion Research online via LexisNexis. [Accession Number: 0273108, 255622]

In this context, racialized perceptions of programs were linked with differential patterns of support for these programs. The relationship between public support for programs and public perceptions regarding the intensity of minority usage of the program is evident in figure 5.3, which examines respondent perceptions of minority usage intensity in combination with support for major cuts to individual programs. The relationship is clear: The greater the public perception that a majority of beneficiaries of a program belong to a racial minority, the greater the support for major cuts to that program.

Welfare provides the most obvious link between racialized perceptions of program beneficiaries and public support. In his 2003 review of seven recent books on welfare, Morone noted that the theme of race "runs quietly" through each: "Every author reviewed here notes that the welfare debates constantly turn on racial images. Race haunts the national discourse on the full range of poor people's programs: drug wars, crime wars, prison construction debates, and the death penalty" (2003, 144). In terms of welfare, "race gets tangled up in perceptions of welfare beneficiaries . . . it dominates popular images of poverty" (2003, 144). The most impressive version of this argument is the work of Martin Gilens—elaborated most fully in *Why Americans Hate Welfare.* Gilens carefully develops a statistical model to predict nonblack opposition to welfare and finds that "racial attitudes are in fact

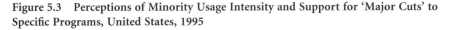

Figure 5.3   Perceptions of Minority Usage Intensity and Support for 'Major Cuts' to Specific Programs, United States, 1995

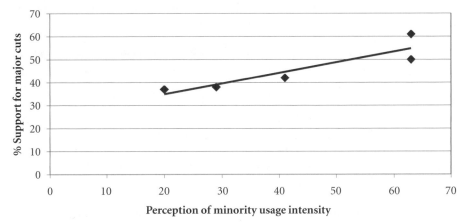

Source: Harvard University and Kaiser Family Foundation, 1995—Questions 107, 108, 109, 113, 115 for support for major cuts by program; Questions 121, 122, 123, 127, 129 for perceptions of minority usage intensity.

the most important source of opposition to welfare among whites" (1995, 994). Racial attitudes (especially regarding the commitment of African Americans to the work ethic) more strongly determine support for welfare and the broader welfare state than other factors, such as self-interest or commitment to principles of individualism or egalitarianism (1995, 995). In turn opposition to welfare has been heightened by racialized perceptions of the welfare beneficiary population that Gilens attributes to racially biased media coverage (1999, 173).

Racial attitudes had important effects in lowering public support for government spending and taxes more generally as well as undermining public support for particular programs in this period. These attitudes might well have been expected to lower public support for health insurance reform—especially reform that extended coverage to the uninsured. As argued below, however, this was not the case.

The Politics of Race and Opportunities for Health Reform

In contrast to the mainstream literature, which has largely ignored the issue of race in relation to the Clinton reforms, a few observers have drawn links between health insurance reform and issues related to race.[7] McDaniel bluntly argues that "anyone who believes that rich white people are prepared to absorb increased costs of medicine for black people is living in a fool's paradise" (1985, 110). In regard specifically to the Clinton health reforms, it has been argued that a "divisive, coded, racial rhetoric emerged" (Morone 1995, 393). Such rhetoric is epitomized by a public official's statement that "you can't expect the hard-working people in suburban Cook County to go into the same health care alliance as the crackheads in Chicago" (Morone 1995, 393).

The most pointed elaboration of the linkage between race and health reform is presented by Richard Iton in his brief examination of the Clinton reforms undertaken in his broader review of the effects of race on the politics of the left in the United States (2000). In Iton's analysis, the most important impact of the politics of race was their effect on public opinion regarding health insurance reform (2000, 153). Central to this argument is the claim that perceptions of the uninsured have taken on a racial cast and, as a corollary, the problem of uninsurance has been understated. Iton argues that a divide has been constructed between the insured and the uninsured with uninsurance being reframed as an "us" versus "them" issue—a construction that he argues "could not be clearer" in terms of its racial coding (2000, 169). Following the type of argument made by Gilens in regard to welfare, Iton argues that "the ability of the antireform interests and the apparent willingness of the media to downplay the gravity of the problems of the uninsured related to racial considerations. The immediate perception was that the completely uninsured were disproportionately nonwhite."[8]

Second, Iton argues that opponents of reform deliberately attempted to undermine public support by constructing a link between health reform and welfare through claims that "significant health care reform was not necessary but another attempt to institute a welfare program" (2000, 167). The ability of opponents to cast health reform as another welfare program, he continues, would "trigger negative responses based on the historical conflation of racial and class understandings and weaken support for any proposed legislation" (169).[9]

The following section, however, argues that the politics of race intersected with the politics of health reform in a much different way than posited by this analysis. Rather than failing because of association with racialized images, health reform proceeded precisely because the structure of existing programs had helped render racial dynamics latent, and it was this characteristic of health reform debates that the Clinton administration desperately tried to preserve while contributing to the racial charging of the American political system with its initiatives on welfare and crime control. Having let the proverbial genie out of the bottle, the Clinton reformers found it difficult to control.

The Relative Popularity of Health Reform

Health care reform was attractive politically precisely because of its relative public popularity, which can be explained, in turn, by its intersection with the politics of race. From 1975 through 1989, public support for government intervention in health policy was greater than public support for government intervention in domestic policy more generally as well as being greater than public support for programs to aid the poor (Schlesinger and Lee 1994, 360). By the late 1980s public support for government intervention in health was higher than had been the case a decade earlier—the only policy area in which public support for government intervention had increased.[10] In two polls in 1990, 72 percent and 73 percent of respondents stated that they supported a national health plan (Blendon and Donelan 1990, 209).

This level of public support for government intervention was related to the fact that health care had not been racialized to the degree evident in other policy areas such as welfare. As Schlesinger and Lee found in their impressive 1994 study, welfare was strongly racially identified in terms of a correlation between support for welfare and concern for the well-being of blacks among all respondents and also in differences between African American and white respondents in support for welfare. In stark contrast, health care was not strongly racially identified (1994, 364). As respondents (both African American and white) became more supportive of "aid to blacks" they became slightly less supportive of government intervention in health policy and "the greater the concern for the well-being of blacks . . . the more support is shifted away from health programs toward redistributive programs and policies" (1994, 354, 359). Similarly, differences between whites and African Americans in supporting government involvement in health were much less marked than differences in support for programs for the poor or for domestic policies in general.[11] While race was the single strongest determinant of support for government involvement in domestic policy generally and programs for the poor, income was a stronger determinant of support for government involvement in health policy than race.

Public Perceptions Regarding the Uninsured

The lack of racialization of health insurance as an issue is linked to the fact that perceptions of the uninsured are not highly racialized. Beginning in 1993 a number of polls asked respondents to describe uninsured Americans using the one or two groups that would come first to the respondent's mind. In two polls taken in 1993 only 13 percent and 19 percent of respondents identified uninsured Americans as belonging to a minority group. In both cases, this response was less popular than a wide range of other responses (ranking as the seventh and fifth most popular responses, respectively) and, in both cases, was a much less common response than identifying the uninsured as "poor people" (44 percent and 48 percent, respectively) or "unemployed" (36 percent and 37 percent, respectively) (Kaiser Foundation and Harvard School of Public Health 1993; Robert Wood Johnson Foundation and Harvard School of Public Health 1993). To the degree that there were racialized perceptions of both the poor and unemployed, these responses might indirectly reflect a racialized perception of the uninsured. Direct evidence of a highly racialized image of the uninsured is limited.

At the same time, public perceptions have significantly overestimated the prevalence of uninsurance. In a poll conducted in 1991 only 12 percent of respondents believed (correctly) that 20 percent of the population or less was uninsured. Twenty-eight percent of respondents estimated the rate of uninsurance of the American population between 20 percent and 30 percent, while fully 57 percent estimated the rate of uninsurance to be above 30 percent—double the actual rate of uninsurance (*CBS News, New York Times* 1991). Consistent with the findings of numerous other polls, this represents a staggering overestimation of the degree of uninsurance.[12] Concomitantly, the greater the perception that uninsurance is widespread, the less likely respondents are to perceive uninsurance as limited to minorities—racial or otherwise.

Not only did public perceptions overestimate the degree of uninsurance, uninsured status was increasingly coming to be seen as problematic. Public perceptions regarding the ability of the poor to access needed medical care dropped substantially over the decade prior to the Clinton reform efforts (Harvey 1993). While nearly half of respondents in 1982 believed that the poor could get needed medical care, this perception declined steadily so that by 1991 only a quarter of respondents believed that the poor could access needed medical services.[13]

This lack of a racialized imagery of the uninsured coupled with overestimation of the degree of uninsurance and a growing appreciation of the problems attendant with the lack of insurance helps explain the political popularity of universal health insurance coverage. As Blendon and Donelan note, "For many years, public opinion surveys have indicated that a majority of Americans (75 to 82 percent) believe government should provide the resources necessary for medical care to be available to everyone who needs it" (1990, 209). In a 1993 poll, 72 percent of recipients stated that coverage of the uninsured was a "very important" goal for national health reform, with an addition 15 percent stating it was a "fairly important" goal (see figure 5.4). Support for universal coverage was not significantly different from concern with addressing the issue of cost control or ensuring the quality of health services.[14] These high levels of support for universal coverage reflect broad public concern for the uninsured.

Figure 5.4   Public Perceptions of the Importance of Various Goals of National Health Reform, 1993

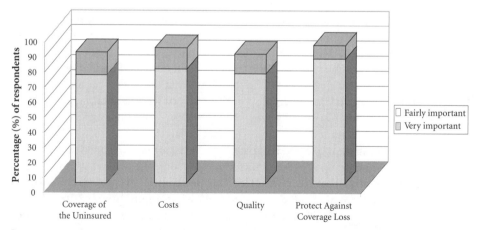

Source:
Robert Wood Johnson Foundation and Harvard School of Public Health. 1993. *American Attitudes Toward Health Care Reform.* 16 May 1993. Accessed from Roper Center for Public Opinion Research online via LexisNexis. [Accession Numbers: 0197066, 0197067, 0197070, 0197071]

Public Perceptions of Medicaid Coverage

Part of the explanation for the weakness of the link in public perceptions between minority status and uninsured status is the perception that African Americans disproportionately receive public health insurance coverage. Racialized perceptions of Medicaid enrollment, for example, could be expected to have the concomitant effect of deracializing perceptions of the uninsured. As outlined in figure 5.3 above, 41 percent of respondents believed that more than half of all Medicaid recipients were composed of members of minority groups. Given these perceptions, it is perhaps less surprising that a majority of respondents (56 percent) in 1989 believed that "because many blacks get free medical care at clinics and through Medicaid, the result they get is as good as whites" while only 39 percent did not believe this claim (NAACP 1989). In a 1999 survey, more respondents believed that blacks were better off (3 percent) or just as well off (46 percent) as whites in terms of having health insurance than those who believed that blacks were worse off (44 percent) in this regard (Kaiser Family Foundation 1999). That nearly 50 percent of respondents did not expect differences between blacks and whites in terms of their health insurance status is highly contrary to the argument that the public overwhelmingly perceives the uninsured population to be predominantly African American.

At the same time, public health insurance programs have also remained relatively insulated from the politics of race. This is especially important in the case of Medicaid, which could be expected to be particularly vulnerable. Political support for Medicaid, it has been argued, has been undermined by its links with the AFDC program: "If the Medicaid program were not seen as part of an unpopular welfare system, public support for expanding the coverage provided for low-income Americans would be stronger" (Blendon and Donelan 1990, 211). Depressed levels of public support for the Medicaid program resulting from its linkage with welfare, to the degree this occurred, could similarly be argued to have an implicitly racial basis—following Gilen's compelling argument that low levels of popular support for AFDC are a result of racially based perceptions of the program's main clientele.

The actual operation and development of the Medicaid program, however, has prevented it from adopting a more highly racialized cast than might have otherwise been the case.[15] Perceptions of minority usage of Medicaid were much lower than might have been expected. For example, the proportion of Medicaid recipients who were black (34 percent in 1995) was comparable to the proportion of Food Stamp recipients who were black (36 percent), yet 63 percent of respondents believed that a majority of Food Stamp recipients were members of minority groups while only 41 percent of respondents believed that a majority of Medicaid recipients were members of minority groups (see figure 5.3). The most likely explanation for such differences is the differential treatment of these programs in the media and by key political and public officials.

Crucially, the construction of Medicaid as a program serving not only low-income people but also the elderly dulled the racial cast of the program. A key element was the inclusion of nursing home care for the elderly alongside the provision of public health insurance for the needy, which fundamentally transformed the dynamics of the program (see especially Grogan and Patashnik 2003a, 2003b). One obvious effect has been to weaken media and political portrayals of Medicaid as a primarily race-based program. Despite the fact that Medicaid disproportionately benefits African Americans and Hispanics, "policy makers rarely cast Medicaid in these terms" (Schlesinger and Lee 1994, 329).

This perception helped insulate the Medicaid program from the politics of race and, in turn, insulated broader health care reform debates from the issue of race. For example, debates about welfare reform—a policy arena where the main public program had a highly racialized public image—could not help but implicate issues related to race. As neither of the two major public health insurance programs had images that were so racialized, debates about health care reform did not automatically raise issues related to race.

The Clinton Strategy

The Clinton reformers were clearly aware of the possibility that health reform could be cast as another effort to provide benefits disproportionately to the poor and that this carried the risk that debates over health reform could be cast in racialized terms. Thus, instead, the main thrust of the reform proposals was to appeal to those who already had health insurance but were underinsured, found insurance too expensive, or were worried about losing insurance if they changed their jobs, lost their jobs or had preexisting conditions (Skocpol 1996, 116–20). An internal memo stated the administration position with blunt precision: "We should not even talk about '37 million uninsured' because this is not who the proposal is designed to protect" (Skocpol 1996, 118). The term "Health Security" was adopted precisely to displace the use of "universal coverage," which might be associated with extending coverage to the poor as opposed to guaranteeing those with coverage that they would not lose it (Hacker 1997, 140). Similarly, the decision to incorporate relatively comprehensive standard benefits in the proposal package was to ensure that guaranteed coverage was not perceived as being primarily aimed at those who did not already have insurance coverage: "The administration's choice to guarantee comprehensive benefits fit closely with Bill Clinton's carefully fashioned political image: He was not a 'traditional Democrat' offering 'welfare' to the 'poor.' He was, instead, a reformed Democrat offering 'security' to the 'middle class'" (Skocpol 1996, 65).

This strategy shifted as the political chances of success began to dim. Brandishing a pen, Clinton confronted Congress in his 1994 State of the Union address vowing to veto any health care proposal that would not provide coverage for everyone. Clinton also made the link between health insurance reform and welfare:

> I know it will be difficult to tackle welfare reform in 1994 at the same time we tackle health care. But let me point out, I think it is inevitable and imperative. It is estimated that one million people are on welfare today because it's the only way they can get health care coverage for their children. Those who choose to leave welfare for jobs without health benefits, and many entry level jobs don't have health benefits, find themselves in the incredible position of paying taxes that help to pay for health care

coverage for those who made the other choice, to stay on welfare. No wonder people leave work and go back to welfare, to get health care coverage. We've got to solve the health care problem to have real welfare reform."[16]

Thus, ironically, attempts to link health reform and welfare—which might have been expected to open up health care reform to political backlash—were made by proponents of reform. Rather than making any attempt to link health reform and welfare, opponents of reform continually emphasized their relatively simple message that there was no crisis in health care requiring the type of radical overhaul proposed by the administration—a position that would ultimately prevail.[17]

The Failure of the Clinton Health Reforms

If one point can be clearly drawn from the voluminous literature on the failure of the Clinton reform, it is surely that this outcome was heavily overdetermined—a large number of causal factors all pushed in the same direction, and uncoupling the individual causal effects of these factors is fraught with peril. Attributing the failure to specific causal factors or, alternatively, asserting the outcome was inevitable strains credulity. Recognizing this, two important contextual factors among the elements contributing to this failure relate to the intersection of the politics of race and public policy. While, as outlined above, the direct effects of race in limiting political support for reform were marginal, the indirect effects were significant.

First, dynamics related to race helped create a context unfavorable to expanding federal services or increasing taxes. As clearly outlined in figure 5.2, concerns about too much spending on minorities played a central role in undermining support generally for expanding services or increasing taxes. The Clinton plan was, if nothing else, widely perceived as an expansion of federal services. On the tax side, the lack of public support for higher taxes, which was also strongly conditioned by concerns about spending on minorities, created a context in which the Clinton administration felt bound to adopt a revenue-neutral approach. Stuck between the proverbial rock and hard place, proposing an increase in taxes would have represented a serious political liability. Yet the plan's failure to specify new revenue sources became an important element in the declining popularity of the Clinton proposals. In the absence of new revenue sources, important constituencies—such as seniors—became convinced that expanding coverage to the uninsured would be financed through cuts to their own coverage (Skocpol 1996).

Second, in the highly race-charged context of the early 1990s to which the Clinton administration itself had contributed through its strong focus on racially identified issues, ending welfare and controlling crime dominated the attention of both the public and policymakers. In turn health insurance, which was much less highly racially identified, dropped in priority. As Blendon and Donelan note, 72 percent of respondents in a poll said they favored a national health care program but only 14 percent identified health care as one of the two most important issues facing the country—in comparison with 64 percent who identified drug use (1990, 209). This was not a propitious context for reform. Health care was included as a plank in the

Clinton campaign and subsequently in his administration's policy program in part because it was insulated from the politics of race. Paradoxically, it would suffer as a political priority for the same reason.

Conclusion

The politics of race played into health care reform in the 1990s in a much different fashion than had been the case in the 1960s, not because the politics of race were no longer salient in shaping public policy debates in the United States but because the configuration of programs that had emerged from the 1960s had shifted the operation of these dynamics as they intersected with the politics of health care. The programs from the 1960s, themselves crucially shaped by the politics of race, created an opportunity to insulate the future politics of health care reform from the direct effects of race that would so significantly shape other policy areas such as welfare. In the highly race-charged atmosphere of the early 1990s, the differing levels of racial identification of these distinct issue areas played an important role in generating an opportunity for health care reform.

At the same time, the conjuncture of the politics of welfare reform, crime control, and health care reform had crucial indirect effects in limiting the likelihood of success of health insurance reforms. Attempts at reform in the first two policy areas ultimately contributed to a general context unfavorable to health care expansion as well as draining political attention away from health insurance reform.[18] The failure of health reform in this period neither compellingly demonstrates that this outcome was inevitable nor conclusively shows that similar reforms would not have been (or could not be) successful in a more favorable political context. Nevertheless, reform failed, and universal health insurance coverage in the United States was not forthcoming. In helping shape this outcome the politics of race contributed to perpetuating the longstanding exceptionalism of the American system relative to those of other industrialized western countries, including its closest neighbor, Canada.

PART III

Public Health Insurance in Canada

CHAPTER SIX

Federal Failure, Provincial Success—Reform in Canada, 1945–49

The evolution of the Canadian system of organizing and paying for health care services has been a long, complex, and stormy struggle, often beset with extraordinary conflict and influenced greatly by the political and economic vicissitudes and crises of this turbulent twentieth century.

Malcolm G. Taylor, *Insuring National Health Care*

Social Medicine is the first step, and a long step, toward the Gehenna of the Welfare State.

William Magner, CMA President, "Health Insurance"

IN THE WORLD WAR II and early postwar period, territorial politics helped shape federal interest in health insurance in Canada but, paradoxically, also set boundaries on the possibilities for national health insurance reform. Federal proposals, as had been the case in the United States in the same period, failed—ultimately as a result of the territorial politics inscribed in the system of Canadian federalism. The federal attempt at reform, however, temporarily relaxed the constraining effects of federalism on provincial-level reform and thus provided a brief window of opportunity for the breakthrough of successful reform in Saskatchewan in 1947.

The Failure of Comprehensive Health Insurance at the Federal Level

The initial push for public health insurance reform in the World War II period took place at the federal level in Canada. Federal proposals in the early 1940s initially contemplated a federally administered system of comprehensive health insurance coverage. Others proposed federal matching grants for provincial provision of public insurance for a similarly comprehensive range of health services. Finally, others recommended leaving health insurance completely to the provinces. The system that emerged roughly fifteen years later was a federal–provincial system limited to hospital insurance that, while setting broad national principles, left administration to the provinces—a system that none of the early proponents of reform had envisioned. In large part, this outcome reflected the degree to which public health insurance reform was intertwined with territorial politics and was the result of a reform process in which successful outcomes were highly tenuous. In contrast with early proposals for reform illustrating the different visions—one federalist and one provincialist—informing proposals for public health insurance reform, more moderate proposals (tilting toward the latter vision) came to dominate but even these initially floundered on the shoals of the territorial politics inscribed in Canadian federal–provincial relations.

Competing Territorial Orientations of Reform

From the initial discussions of health insurance reform in the late 1930s and early 1940s, all the major proposals for reform envisioned public health insurance coverage for a comprehensive range of medical services. Despite this basic similarity, proposals were split into two camps dominated by different visions of the territorial orientation of reforms—a federalist vision and provincialist vision. The former envisioned a single national program of public health insurance administered by the federal government while the latter envisioned a national system of provincial programs—in some versions, developed with the aid of federal financial contributions. These different visions highlighted the territorially based political tensions underpinning health insurance reform in Canada.

The Centralist Vision

In the World War II period, a single federal program of national public health insurance seemed a realistic possibility. There was no doubt that health care was an area of primarily provincial jurisdiction; however, the exigencies of the Great Depression and World War II had resulted in considerable centralization of the Canadian federation. In social policy, a constitutional amendment allowing for the federal assumption of provincial jurisdiction over unemployment insurance was passed in the early 1940s—a constitutional development that recurred in the early 1950s for universal noncontributory pensions and in the mid-1960s for contributory pensions. A similar initiative in health services was contemplated in the early 1940s at the highest reaches of government by the Economic Advisory Committee of Cabinet, chaired by the deputy minister of finance.

War had an important impact on public health insurance policy as it did in other social policy fields and other countries. It was, according to some observers, the "strongest impetus" to the development of public health insurance in Canada (Taylor 1990, 33). World War II had been a critical catalyst to health insurance reform debates in the United States by highlighting the poor health status of service-aged men, as had also been the case in Canada. In Canada, World War II also played an important role both in raising faith in government (which under considerable levels of centralization had successfully managed the war effort) as well as "illuminat[ing] the possibilities of recreating a society that was more humane, caring, and compassionate" (Taylor 1990, 33).

The most critical domestic issue raised by the war, however, was the second conscription crisis in Canada—an issue with a sharply territorial orientation. Deep divisions between Québec and the rest of Canada on the issue of a mandatory military draft resurfaced. In early 1942 a national referendum allowing for the possibility of conscription was held. The referendum received majority support in all provinces outside Québec (with an 80 percent approval rating) while in Québec 73 percent voted against it. When the federal government passed a bill allowing (but not requiring) conscription, riots broke out in Montréal.[1]

This second conscription crisis highlighted the degree to which the Québec population still did not feel a strong attachment to the national government as well as the degree to which the federal government had failed after the first conscription crisis to create direct connections with this segment of the Canadian population. Direct federal intervention in social policy, including areas such as unemployment insurance, old age pensions, and health insurance, could provide a powerful tool for the federal government to touch the lives of Canadian citizens directly and strengthen the bonds to the national government and Canadian society more generally. A federal program of health insurance had the potential to play a key role in territorial integration.

Federal leaders saw Québec as already having embarked on a campaign to alter the terms of confederation by reinterpreting and expanding its autonomous powers. Federal officials believed that a conflict with Québec over the terms of reconstruction was inevitable (Taylor 1978, 44). They were also acutely aware that a majority of Québécois voters would support their provincial government in a conflict with the federal government because, as Prime Minister St. Laurent put it, "people were made constantly aware of the services which provincial governments rendered while they tended to think of the central government as the one imposing the burdens such as taxation and conscription" (Taylor 1978, 44). Measures such as family allowances (to provide families with children a monthly payment direct from the federal government) were expressly designed to "correct" what federal political leadership saw as this imbalance. Health insurance was also subject to this political calculation.

The Provincialist Vision

The provincialist vision had found expression in the reports of several appointed commissions. The Royal Commission on Dominion–Provincial Relations (Rowell–Sirois commission) argued that, unlike old-age security and unemployment insurance, health insurance should remain a provincial responsibility.[2] The report had an overall provincialist bent philosophically and was an early example in Canada of applying the principle of subsidiarity—leaving functions to the lowest level of government capable of performing them effectively.[3] The rationale offered for straight federal programs of unemployment insurance and contributory pensions was that provinces would be unlikely to undertake such programs; provinces needed to maintain their industries' competitive positions and there were administrative difficulties with workers moving between provinces. These issues were not seen as problematic enough in the case of public health insurance to warrant federal assumption of responsibility in this area.[4]

The central argument made for maintaining primary provincial jurisdiction over health was the integration of health services: "The desirability of coordinating all medical services within the province under provincial control is a strong argument against the establishment of any scheme which would remove any large group within the province from provincial responsibility, as a Dominion health insurance scheme would do" (Royal Commission on Dominion–Provincial Relations 1939, 42). At the same time, the Royal Commission was highly skeptical of conditional grants—believing them to be politically unenforceable.[5] Therefore it recommended leaving health insurance entirely to the provinces.

For pragmatic reasons this position was partly echoed in the report of the Heagerty committee, which the federal government had appointed in 1942 to study the issue of health insurance and, in less than year, produced a blueprint for a national program of health insurance.[6] The Heagerty report rejected both a federally administered program as well as simply leaving health insurance to the provinces and, instead, favored conditional grants in aid. The report certainly foresaw some significant degree of uniformity among the provinces and included model legislation for provincial health insurance plans.[7] The Heagerty committee's position was based not on a philosophical predisposition toward a provincially administered system (as had animated the Rowell–Sirois commission) but rather on political pragmatism: "It became clear that there was no possibility of achieving unanimous agreement of the provinces to a constitutional amendment transferring health services administration and financing to the federal government" (Taylor 1990, 15). Furthermore, the realpolitik of the situation was clear. From the provincial perspective, being relieved of financial responsibility for the unemployed (not a politically powerful or popular group) was a politically attractive alternative. Giving up responsibility for the provision of health services certainly did not hold the same attraction (Taylor 1990, 15).

Indeed the political reality governing health care provision in the provinces was more complex than was the case for unemployment insurance and contributory pensions (neither of which existed in the provinces). Although no province at the time had a program of public health insurance, a federal program of health insurance nevertheless had the potential to disrupt existing arrangements governing the provision of health services in the provinces—most notably in Québec. The political status quo that had emerged in Québec was an arrangement by which the Québécois political elite managed an entente between an Anglophone business elite that largely controlled the economy and the Catholic Church, which largely governed Québec society. The church assumed many of the functions of the state, including the provision of education, welfare, and through the maintenance of religious hospitals, health care. Church control of these functions was seen as a critical element in the overall preservation of Québécois society and, by extension, French existence in North America. Federal interference in health care—especially through a federally administered program of public health insurance—would have posed a significant challenge to these well-established social arrangements, much as federal intervention in the United States threatened to disrupt established social arrangements in the South. The provincial government could insist on its constitutionally granted jurisdictional prerogatives to preserve the integrity of these arrangements—making significant federal intrusion into the field politically untenable.

Cognizant of such distinctiveness, the Royal Commission argued that it was "essential that . . . responsibility for providing medical and hospital services and the choice of means should be left to the provinces" not only because of social and economic differences among the provinces but also because of great differences between them in "social outlook" (1939, 42). The Royal Commission believed not only that these regional differences in Canada precluded a politically acceptable national program but also that centralization of jurisdiction over health, in the face of "pronounced regional differences in social philosophy" would not be conducive to "national unity in general" (1939, 34). How much provincial diversity was required to maintain national unity and, in turn, how much diversity national unity could withstand reflected a perennial question central to territorial integration in Canada. The commonality the provincialist vision shared with its centralist counterpart was that both saw the matter of health insurance, in large part, in terms of its importance for national unity.

The Failure of the Dominion–Provincial Conference on Reconstruction

While the federal government ultimately settled on a compromise between the polar extremes of a straight federal program and leaving health insurance entirely to the provinces, the final proposal rested somewhat closer to the provincialist version.

The federalist version had emerged most clearly after the Heagerty proposals, and accompanying draft legislation (prior to its public release) was presented to the cabinet and subsequently referred to the Economics Advisory Committee in 1943 (Taylor 1990, 48). In sharp contrast to the Heagerty proposals, the committee recommended that health insurance be financed and administered on a strictly federal basis, as was unemployment insurance, recognizing that this would require a constitutional amendment. The cabinet was not persuaded but agreed to appoint a special committee of House of Commons to examine the issue of health insurance.

By 1945, in the face of an impending federal election, the federal government had backed away even from the Heagerty proposals to make public health insurance a more politically attractive component of a larger package for postwar reconstruction. Doing so required making the proposals "less interventionist" (Taylor 1990, 53). To this end the new federal proposals abandoned the idea of a model bill for the provinces and avoided specifying any method of provincial financing. With this package of proposals in hand, an election was called for June 1945 in which health insurance became a major issue and, with strong public support, was endorsed by all four political parties.[8]

After securing reelection, the Liberal government included public health insurance reform as part of the broader package of "Green Book Proposals" for postwar reconstruction in 1945. The federal government, at the Dominion–Provincial Conference on Post-War Reconstruction of 1945, offered grants-in-aid for medical, hospital, dental, pharmaceutical, and nursing benefits. The terms of the proposals were very open-ended, and "the original plan for national legislation in the interests of promoting national uniformity and adequacy had been dropped" (Guest 1997, 132).

The government of Québec rejected the social insurance proposals. Other elements of the overall package also met with serious provincial resistance.[9] Despite the softening of federal proposals as outlined above, the Québec premier opposed federal proposals on the basis that they were "incompatible with the autonomy of the province" and "would inevitably lead to Federal interference in all these fields which ought to be free of Dominion authority."[10] Of course, the provincial government had no plans of its own to enter the public health insurance field; rather, it was protecting existing arrangements in which the Catholic Church had largely assumed the responsibility for providing the province's health services. The provincial government was not willing to be subjected to the political pressure that would have undoubtedly been generated by a federal cost-sharing program. Nor was it willing, on principle, to cede the initiative to federal social policy in an area of provincial jurisdictional competence. As a result of the inability to achieve federal–provincial consensus on this and other issues, the "entire package was jettisoned and the first significant plan for a comprehensive medical care system in Canada was stillborn" (Guest 1997, 132).

Despite the failure of the 1945 reconstruction proposals, the one part of the package to be salvaged was a provision for health grants. The 1948 National Health Grants Program provided federal grants to the provinces for a range of health-related activities. By far the most significant of these were matching grants for hospital construction similar to federal grants for hospital construction adopted in the United States in the same year, with initial provincial recommendations for such grants being expressly based on legislation before the U.S. Congress (Taylor 1978, 60).

Repercussions

Three major repercussions resulted from the failure of the federal health insurance proposals. The first, outlined more fully in the following section, was the impact on public health insurance reforms already under way in the provinces. Second, the failure signaled to the medical profession that public health insurance in Canada was vulnerable. Organized medicine responded by formally shifting to an explicit policy of opposition to public health insurance. Third, the failure of the proposals at this juncture pushed health insurance reforms into a period in which they would no longer have the support, at the federal level, of the leadership of the governing Liberal party.

In the initial discussions between the federal government and various stakeholder groups, the CMA had been willing to cooperate in the formulation of a public health insurance plan. The CMA, in the past, had vacillated on the issue, and the BCMA (with the tacit support of the CMA) had strongly opposed public health insurance in British Columbia in the 1930s. As a result, their support of federal public health insurance proposals (along with that of the Canadian Hospital Association and the Canadian Life Insurance Association [CLIA]) was to the "surprise of many" (Taylor 1990, 49). This support was more tactical than philosophical, and "the elected representatives of organized medicine in Canada were fully reconciled to, if not enthusiastic about, a new system of medical care financing which, they anticipated, would have a major impact on medical practice" (Taylor 1990, 51; see also Naylor 1986, 122). The CMA viewed federal reform as an opportunity to pursue its goals—especially in regard to asserting physician control over any resulting public health insurance plan—in a single federal venue rather than on nine separate provincial fronts.[11]

In a changed political context, physician support for public health insurance evaporated. As had been the case in British Columbia, the enthusiasm of the medical profession cooled as the outlines of a plan became more substantial. While in early 1943, there was "an overall readiness to work within a public sector framework," this readiness "attenuated gradually over the next eighteen months" (Naylor 1986, 111). Shortly after the federal proposals for national public health insurance failed, the CMA reversed its support for public health insurance and endorsed voluntary plans, with the government ensuring broad coverage by subsidizing premiums for those with low income (Taylor 1990, 84).[12] The AMA later mirrored this position. The 1949 presidential address to the CMA was as clear a statement against public health insurance as anything emanating from the AMA:

> Socialized Medicine means a crushing burden on the taxpayer. Social Medicine means a harassed medical profession, deprived of all that now attracts clever and highminded men and women to a medical career. Socialized medicine means an inferior medical service, staffed, in time, by inferior men. Social Medicine is the first step, and a long step, toward the Gehenna of the Welfare State. (Magner 1949, 196)

As had been the case in British Columbia in the late 1930s and in the United States, hospital and medical associations as well as private insurance companies "leaped into the vacuum of unfulfilled expectations" following the collapse of the reconstruction proposals for health insurance (Taylor 1990, 60). Various plans were offered (including Blue Cross and Blue Shield plans), and the growth of these plans was impressive.[13] While coverage varied across provinces, by 1952 two-thirds of the population in Ontario (a province representing roughly one-third of the Canadian population) was covered by voluntary hospital insurance (Taylor 1990, 66).

The development of these private plans had crucial impacts on the development of public health insurance in Canada. But the voluntary insurance plans in Canada did not preclude the development of public health insurance, as is often argued to have been the case in the United States. They did, however, have a crucial and lasting effect, as they had in the United States, entrenching fee-for-service payment and private medical practice. After the expansion of voluntary insurance and prepayment plans, "a salaried state medical service . . . was even less feasible politically;

nor was it likely that state medical care insurance could be organized around capitation payments for [general practitioners]" (Naylor 1986, 172).

As with the medical profession, the position of the senior leadership of the governing Liberal party also shifted. Mackenzie King, who had first committed the Liberal Party to national health insurance in 1919 and had been prime minister since 1935, was replaced by Louis St. Laurent as leader of the Liberal Party in 1948. In the 1949 election, St. Laurent avoided making any firm commitment on the issue of health insurance, and although the party platform reaffirmed the party's commitment to health insurance, the issue played a minor role in the Liberal campaign.[14] Following its election victory the federal Liberals abandoned their commitment to health insurance. This is not surprising considering St. Laurent's philosophy regarding the appropriate role of government was in stark opposition to such intervention. St. Laurent "believed in free enterprise" and "government action to bring about a universal program of health insurance that would have the effect of removing the field from private enterprise would fit most uncomfortably within such philosophic parameters" (Taylor 1990, 83).

Conclusions

Territorial politics—especially the need for the federal government to reinforce its connection with individual citizens in Québec in the wake of the second conscription crisis—helped place the issue of a national system of health insurance on the political agenda in the early 1940s. While a national program of public health insurance could serve this territorially integrative function, it also threatened to disrupt existing social relations in Québec, and not surprisingly, Québec insisted on its jurisdictional prerogative to forestall federal intervention in this field. This failure to achieve a national program of public health insurance meant that the next round of national health insurance reform had to wait for over a decade and had to be fashioned in a much less politically hospitable climate marked by the growing resistance of the medical profession and political leadership much less predisposed toward public health insurance than had been the case in 1945. By pushing the timing back, the failure endangered the very prospect of national health insurance in Canada and helped ensure that the next round of reforms were limited to the much narrower issue of hospital insurance.

Reform in the Canadian Provinces, 1947–56

One of the most important outcomes of this failure was its contribution to the main breakthrough in public health insurance that occurred in Saskatchewan right after the war. The reform, which was largely an accident of historical circumstances, occurred because the pending federal–provincial cost-sharing program under the reconstruction plan temporarily suspended the dynamics constraining provinces from going it alone. In turn the success of reform in Saskatchewan contributed to the advent of hospital insurance in British Columbia in 1949. Contrary to the expectations of certain path-dependent analyses, these reforms took place despite the fact that these provinces already had programs of comprehensive medical care for social assistance recipients and, in the case of British Columbia, had been subject to an aggressive campaign on the part of organized medicine to forestall public health insurance reform through promoting voluntary health insurance plans—conditions that, according to arguments outlined in chapter 2 might have been expected to block public health insurance reforms.[15]

Hospital Insurance in Saskatchewan

The story of the emergence of public hospital insurance in Saskatchewan in this period is more complex and nuanced than is often portrayed. Public health insurance did not emerge simply as the natural result of a government with a socialist public philosophy holding power in a parliamentary system. The outcome was far more contingent than such an interpretation suggests and dependent on the perception—mistaken though it was—that a federal program for cost-sharing health insurance was imminent.

Necessity as the Mother of Reform

Various government programs in the hospital and medical-care sectors had developed incrementally over a long time in Saskatchewan—less as a matter of ideological predisposition than as a response to necessity. First allowed under provincial legislation in 1916, Saskatchewan had, in various localities, municipal doctor arrangements by which physicians in rural municipalities were paid a stipend by the municipality to supplement their fee-for-service income (Houston 2002, 23).[16] This was seen as a pragmatic response to an immediate problem—the difficulty of retaining physicians in sparsely populated agricultural areas especially during economic downturns that, in a one-crop agricultural economy subject to drought and other natural hazards and based on world commodity prices, were not infrequent.[17]

The Depression and its aftermath provided a strong impetus for some government intervention to provide health services in Saskatchewan. In a survey of ninety rural physicians in the early 1940s, the response was "almost unanimous in declaring that private practice was no longer feasible" (Houston 2002, 36). One particular reply captures the urgency of the mood of rural physicians: "Any system is to be preferred to the present. Collections appear hopeless. I do not know how medical men can hope to carry on out here under present and future conditions" (Houston 2002, 36).[18]

In keeping with the existing pattern of local development, universal hospital and medical insurance first came into being on a regional rather than provincial basis. The Swift Current area in southwestern Saskatchewan was drought stricken and facing serious doctor shortages (Houston 2002, 82). As the private health care system faltered, some sort of public plan appeared to be a necessity. By special legislation, the Swift Current Health Region was created, and universal medical and hospital care was implemented in the region in mid-1946—half a year before universal hospital insurance would be offered across the province. Physician support for such an initiative was split between rural doctors, some of whom believed that they could not continue to practice under existing conditions, and urban doctors, who did not share the plight of their rural colleagues. Physicians in the province's two urban areas, Regina and Saskatoon, "looked askance at this experiment in 'socialized medicine'" (Houston 2002, 84).

These early programs of government intervention in the provision of health services had resulted in public opinion that was favorably predisposed toward public health insurance and led the Saskatchewan College of Physicians and Surgeons as well as the Saskatchewan Association of Rural Municipalities to endorse public hospital insurance (Taylor 1978, 79).

The Role of the Cooperative Commonwealth Federation

It is tempting to assume that since a provincial hospitalization program was implemented after the election of the Cooperative Commonwealth Federation (CCF) in 1944 that it was implemented as a result of that election.[19] The reality is again more complex. As argued above, necessity placed health care on the political agenda. The proposals for health insurance reform at the federal level provided a template for reform as well as the likelihood of future federal cost-sharing. The Liberal government in Saskatchewan in 1944 had already adopted enabling legislation to allow for Saskatchewan's participation in a federal health insurance program before the CCF's election (Naylor 1986, 129).

Hospital insurance proposals that emerged under the Liberals prior to the CCF's election placed public provision on a social insurance basis (e.g., requiring contributory premiums) and limited its provision to hospitals. These design decisions came from an abiding belief on the part of Saskatchewan policymakers that a federal cost-sharing program was imminent. The Select Special Committee on Social Security, which had been appointed by the governing Saskatchewan Liberals, had considered both direct state provision of medical services as well as public health insurance but concluded that "since federal assistance was a prerequisite to the adoption of a scheme of health services in Saskatchewan, and inasmuch as the Dominion government would probably determine which of the two systems it would support, the choice for Saskatchewan was not theirs to make" (Taylor 1978, 76). The Liberal government came to the same conclusion—a plan in Saskatchewan required prior action by the federal government. The Liberals passed enabling legislation for public health insurance that allowed the province to implement a health insurance plan as soon as a federal program was announced (Taylor 1978, 77).

In contrast to these tentative proposals for hospital insurance, the CCF was firmly committed to socialized health services and had been since the Great Depression. In its Regina Manifesto of 1933, the CCF called for "socialized" health services. Health, hospital, and medical services would be "publicly organized"—moving health services from the existing system based on private enterprise to making such services freely available on the same basis as education—the same principle underpinning proposals in the state of New York in 1939 (CCF 1933).[20] The 1944 CCF campaign under T. C. "Tommy" Douglas focused on the issue of health services but argued that health insurance akin to that proposed by the Heagerty committee would be inadequate (Naylor 1986, 137).

Immediately after being elected in 1944 the Douglas government appointed a health commission under Henry Sigerist, a professor of medical history at Johns Hopkins University (Houston 2002, 69). Following the recommendations of the Sigerist report, the province first moved to provide comprehensive health care for social assistance recipients, pensioners, and widows on a fee-for-service basis (Houston 2002, 72). The plan was in operation by January 1, 1945, and provided medical, hospital, and dental care and pharmaceuticals on a means-tested basis for recipients of Old Age Assistance and social assistance (Taylor 1954, 751–52).

At the same time, the government began making plans for universal hospital insurance. As had been the case under the Liberals, the CCF considered it essential that the hospital insurance plan be designed to meet federal requirements (Taylor 1987, 98).[21] It jettisoned its commitment to socialized health services and, instead, adopted the approach that had been initiated under the former Liberal government—universal premium-based insurance limited to hospital services.

Strategic Miscalculation

The Dominion–Provincial Conference on Reconstruction had been launched but not concluded when the Saskatchewan government decided to move ahead with hospital insurance (Taylor 1978, 69). Believing that having a public health insurance program up and running successfully before the next election would be crucial to their reelection, the Saskatchewan officials proceeded with the hospital insurance initiative and took "the gamble to introduce the program before the federal policy had been decided upon" (Taylor 1990, 72–73). The Saskatchewan government, of course, could not know that the federal–provincial negotiations would break down and that federal cost-sharing would, as a result, not be available for another dozen years.[22] As it stood, the provincial government was now publicly committed to instituting a hospital insurance program, and province-wide universal hospitalization insurance became available on January 1, 1947. Given the belief that federal support was essential, the Saskatchewan government would certainly not have proceeded with the hospital insurance plan had it realized that no federal cost-sharing would be forthcoming for more than a decade. The expectation of federal cost-sharing temporarily suspended the constraining dynamics typically faced by provinces attempting to implement major social programs on their own.

The crucial contribution of the CCF government in Saskatchewan in this period was not to be the first provincial government to seriously pursue reform (which the government of British Columbia had done a decade earlier) or to be the only provincial government to undertake reforms (as discussed below, British Columbia adopted a program of social assistance medical care at the same time as Saskatchewan and would implement universal hospital insurance two years after Saskatchewan) or even to be the originator of the idea of public health insurance (in this period forceful impetuses for reform existed in Ottawa including, for example, the Heagerty committee, which had a great influence on debates in Saskatchewan).

Rather, the major contribution of the CCF government was to follow through with the implementation of its hospital insurance program even after its strategic miscalculation in regard to federal cost-sharing became clear. Despite the serious setback represented by the failure of the Conference on Reconstruction to produce cost-sharing, the Saskatchewan government implemented hospital insurance in an administratively effective and politically adroit manner—providing an impressive example that every single other provincial government sent a delegation to Saskatchewan to study. Had the Saskatchewan government wavered or, alternatively, been less successful in its implementation of hospital insurance (as would later be the case in British Columbia), the historical development of public health insurance in Canada would undoubtedly have taken a significantly different path.

Hospital Insurance in British Columbia

In 1947 British Columbia followed Saskatchewan's lead with the governing Liberal–Conservative party deciding to implement a province-wide system of compulsory hospital insurance. Legislation was passed in 1948 and the program scheduled to start on January 1, 1949 (Taylor 1990, 76). The advent of hospital insurance in British Columbia illustrates three important points.

First, public health insurance reform was not solely the prerogative of socialist third parties. Centrist, liberal-dominated governments had undertaken a major push for public health insurance reform from 1935 to 1937.[23] The next attempt at reform, in which provincial hospital insurance was implemented, was undertaken by a Liberal–Conservative coalition that had, in the 1945 election, garnered 56 percent of the popular vote and thirty-seven of forty-eight seats.[24] Second, in British Columbia, a provincial program of comprehensive medical care for social assistance recipients had been in place since 1945 and had not undermined the demand for universal hospital insurance. Third, as outlined in chapter 2, British Columbia had experienced a sustained and vigorous campaign for over a decade by the medical profession to provide voluntary hospital and medical care insurance plans to displace public insurance; however, this did not forestall the advent of public health insurance.

Unlike the case of hospital insurance in Saskatchewan, the BC system had serious administrative problems (Taylor 1990, 76–77). As a result, hospital insurance was the central issue of the 1952 election that resulted in the defeat of the government. The main root of the problems was the system of premium collection, which was abolished in 1954 and was replaced by an increased retail sales tax (Taylor 1990, 78).

Public Health Insurance Reform in the Canadian Provinces and the United States

The success of provincial public health insurance reforms in the late 1940s and 1950s is a key element in numerous interpretations of the divergent trajectories of public health insurance development in Canada and the United States (Hacker 1998; Maioni 1998; Tuohy 1999). Various writers argue that provincial innovations have been crucial in precipitating federal intervention in Canada, eventually leading to a national system of public health insurance—an argument that the following chapter challenges. This debate nevertheless raises the crucial question of why, in the wake of failure to implement reform at the federal level in the immediate post-war period in both countries, provincial experimentation occurred in Canada but did not occur at the state level in the United States (Boase 1996, 18; Hacker 1998, 72; Tuohy 1999, 45).

One potential answer lies in the differential effects of the institution of federalism in the two countries, including the "opportunities federalism created for regional political movements supportive of reform to gain power" (Hacker 1998, 101). How-ever, this interpretation fails to explain why initial attempts at health insurance reforms emerged earlier and on a more widespread basis in the American states than in the Canadian provinces.

A second argument is that fiscal equalization "mitigated provincial fears of labor and capital flight and permitted the poorer provinces to play a leadership role in Canadian social policy that their limited fiscal resources might otherwise have pre-cluded" (Hacker 1998, 73). In this interpretation, the lack of a system of fiscal equalization in the United States helps explain why reforms were not successful in American states as they were in the Canadian provinces. The main problem with this argument is that a program of equalization did not exist until well after the initial implementation of public hospital insurance in Saskatchewan, British Columbia, and Alberta.[25]

A final potential answer is that this pattern was a result of the strategic judgment of reformers. Tuohy argues that the explanation for this difference lies "in the realm of institutions and policy legacies" (1999, 47). Canadian reformers did not have a "singular example of success at the federal level comparable to the American New Deal" and, as a result, were less likely to look to the federal government for social policy reform (1999, 47). At the same time, in the New Deal era, the states—especially those in the South—had come to be seen by reformers in the United States as resistant to social policy reform. Reformers looked to the federal govern-ment as the most propitious route to reform (Tuohy 1999, 48). This interpretation ignores the widespread efforts at state-level reform in the 1940s illustrated, for example, by the serious efforts at reform in California.

In contrast to these arguments, which emphasize the different effects of federal-ism in the two countries, federalism had a similarly dampening effect on state and provincial social policy reforms in both nations. The examples of reform in Califor-nia and British Columbia in the 1930s and early 1940s highlight the difficulty of states or provinces implementing health insurance on their own. It is not surprising that U.S. reformers largely gave up on state-level reforms when it became clear in the late 1940s that a federal program would not be forthcoming. State-level reforms were simply not likely to succeed in the absence of federal reform. At the same time, the major breakthrough in public health insurance in Canada took place because the governing party in Saskatchewan mistakenly anticipated that a federal program would be set up. In turn, the adoption of public hospital insurance reform in British Columbia two years later rested heavily, both politically and administratively, on the example of policy success in Saskatchewan.

The failure of reform in American states and the success of reform in the Canadian provinces was, most clearly, a function of the prospects for reform at the federal level. In the United States after 1948 it seemed relatively clear that the politics of race ensured that a federal program of cost-sharing of universal health insurance would not be forthcoming—effectively forestalling state-level experimentation. Until the territorial politics inscribed in Canadian federalism cut this development short, it appeared that federal intervention in Canada was imminent—precipitating premature province-level reform.

Conclusions

Both the efforts to undertake health insurance reform at the federal level and their failure were deeply conditioned by the politics of territorial integration in Canada and the federal–provincial processes through which these dynamics played out. Public health insurance provided federal policymakers with an opportunity to reinforce notions of national citizenship while these attempts to intrude on existing social arrangements—most notably in the province of Québec—generated provincial resistance to federal reform efforts. In this sense, the circumstances surrounding failure of federal-level reform closely mirrored those in the United States. In both cases, sectional interests (in the South and in Québec, respectively) opposed federal intervention in social policy broadly and in public health insurance more specifically, using crucial institutional levers (control of congressional committees by southern elected representatives in the United States and aggressive protection of jurisdictional authority by the provincial government of Québec in Canada) to protect existing social relations within the region (segregation in the South and the Catholic Church's dominance over social arrangements in Québec). In both cases, the outcome at the federal level was, at least for the time being, the same.

In Canada, however, failure had a crucial legacy—the spawning of universal public hospital insurance in Saskatchewan. As argued in earlier chapters, it was not the case that the constraining dynamics of federalism operated differently in Canada than in the United States but, rather, that the circumstances surrounding the failure of federal health insurance reforms in Canada temporarily suspended the operation of these dynamics. The emergence of public hospital insurance in this brief window of opportunity was nothing if not contingent.

There is little doubt that under slightly different circumstances—such as the province anticipating the failure of a federal–provincial program due to Québec's intransigence—provincial hospital insurance reforms in Saskatchewan would probably not have not been undertaken. Alternatively, having been undertaken, they simply could have failed as was almost the case in British Columbia. In either case such developments might well have placed public health insurance in Canada on a radically different path than the one it took. At the same time, as argued below, the success of hospital insurance reform in Saskatchewan hardly guaranteed the success of universal public insurance at the federal level. In yet another round of highly contingent reform developments, these themes of territory, national unity, and provincial autonomy again played themselves out in the development of public health insurance in Canada.

CHAPTER SEVEN

National Public Hospital Insurance and Medical Care Insurance in Saskatchewan, 1950–62

I think it would be a most happy solution if the medical profession would assume the administration of and responsibility for a scheme that would provide prepaid medical attention to any Canadian who needed it.

Prime Minister Louis St. Laurent

The concept of universal medical coverage is not new and the approach by government to seek support is just the same as it was when first enunciated by Karl Marx in his Communistic Theories of the last century.

Saskatchewan Medical Association, Public Relations Kit, 1960

THE ADVENT OF HOSPITAL INSURANCE at the provincial level did not automatically translate into the successful implementation of a hospital insurance program at the federal level. Instead, the failure of the federal–provincial negotiations in 1945 pushed subsequent reforms at the federal level into a period where they would have to be undertaken without the support of the medical profession and, as outlined in the following section, under political leadership considerably less predisposed toward direct public intervention in the health insurance field. Neither the federal government nor the Ontario government—whose agreement was key to the adoption of a federal plan—was enthusiastic about the prospect of public intervention in the health insurance field. Despite provincial precedents, the outcome remained far from assured and subject to the vagaries of the politics of Canadian federalism.

Nevertheless, as a result of federal–provincial dynamics, the federal government and Ontario provincial government became caught up in a game of one-upmanship driven by electoral pressures—the result of which was the hospital insurance program, which still constitutes one of two major planks of Canadian medicare today. A number of characteristics of the emergent system now seen as representative of the philosophical underpinnings of health care in Canada (such as universality and first-dollar coverage) came about as pragmatic responses to the immediate administrative problems of implementing a federal–provincial program.

One major consequence of federal cost-sharing for hospital insurance was to set the stage for the inception, four years later, of public insurance for physician care in Saskatchewan. Medical care insurance faced vociferous opposition in Saskatchewan from the medical profession, business, the media, and significant segments of the public—echoing earlier debates over public health insurance in the United States. However, in this case, reform would ultimately be successful.

National Hospital Care Insurance in Canada

In comparison with 1945, none of the key protagonists by the early 1950s—including the prime minister and federal government, the Ontario government, and the CMA—was keen on the idea of public health insurance. St. Laurent as leader of the Liberal Party was clearly not predisposed toward public health insurance although the Liberal cabinet was deeply split philosophically. On the other side of this debate, Paul Martin Sr., as minister of health, was a strong proponent of national health insurance and, over the period that hospital insurance was debated in the federal government, his support and influence in the cabinet grew (Taylor 1987, 128). At the provincial level, the governing Conservatives in Ontario were committed to the principles of free enterprise and limited government, and many individual members of the government were ardent opponents of government health insurance (Taylor 1987, 110, 118–19).

Hospital insurance was caught up in a game of federal–provincial buck-passing and one-upmanship that ultimately resulted in a federal program of hospital insurance. The opening move was the inclusion in the 1953 federal Liberal election platform of a provision (reflecting only lukewarm support for a program of compulsory health insurance) that placed the onus for any further development on the provinces: "The Liberal party is committed to support a policy of contributory health insurance to be administered by the provinces when most of the provinces are ready to join in a nationwide scheme" (Taylor 1990, 84). The rationale was that the federal government should not levy taxes on all Canadian taxpayers to finance benefits provided only in some provinces. If, as the federal government insisted, federal intervention required the agreement of a sufficient number of provinces to represent a majority of the population, the onus rested on Ontario, as Québec had already signaled that it was adamantly opposed to federal incursions in this area of provincial jurisdiction.

This, however, created a catch-22 with both the federal and Ontario governments claiming that other had to move first for health care reform to occur. Under pressure from the legislative opposition, media, and public to do something in regard to health insurance, the Ontario Conservative government claimed that it wished to move on health insurance but doing so would require federal participation. The provincial Liberals and CCF had strongly supported public health insurance in the election of 1951 and would undoubtedly do so again in 1955 (Taylor 1987, 116). In

March of 1955 with a provincial election looming, Premier Leslie Frost again deflected responsibility for health insurance, arguing that, because of lack of federal support, it was impossible (Taylor 1987, 123). In response, prominent federal Liberal Jack Pickersgill argued publicly in Ontario in April—just weeks before the provincial election—that the initiation of a federal public health insurance program would first require the defeat of the Frost government in Ontario (Taylor 1987, 208). The pressure that each government was placing on the other was beginning to mount.

The upcoming federal–provincial conference to renegotiate existing tax agreements provided the Ontario government with a strategic opportunity to demonstrate strong leadership in the arena of health insurance without actually having to commit itself to undertaking a provincial program. The Ontario government, at a federal–provincial meeting to determine the agenda for the conference, pushed hard for the inclusion of health insurance (Taylor 1987, 126). St. Laurent strongly resisted, but his own health minister, Paul Martin Sr., threatened to resign if health insurance was not included on the agenda (Taylor 1990, 89). Finally, the prime minister gave in. Frost could take credit for putting the issue on the federal–provincial agenda in the face of a reluctant federal government.[1]

Having won the election in June 1955 with a comfortable margin, Frost proposed at the federal–provincial conference in October that the federal and provincial governments move forward together on hospital insurance and presented specific proposals centered on a program of hospital care insurance (Taylor 1987, 90). At the conclusion of the conference, a committee on health insurance comprising officials from both levels of government was appointed to study the issue of health insurance (Taylor 1990, 90). The situation did not look particularly propitious for compulsory insurance. At least half the provinces had already signaled a preference for voluntary plans. Furthermore, neither the federal government nor the Ontario government was predisposed toward compulsory public insurance. Frost met with St. Laurent three months later in January 1956: "After the Ontario Premier had left, St. Laurent emerged from his office, and commented in a bemused tone: 'You know, Mr. Frost doesn't like hospital insurance either'" (Taylor 1987, 187).

Nevertheless, under the aegis of the federal minister of health, a federal proposal for a federal–provincial hospital insurance plan was presented at a committee meeting in early 1956. The proposal would again require the implementation of programs in a majority of provinces with a majority of the population—meaning, in effect, that Ontario would have to agree since Québec's opposition was already anticipated. Ontario had strong objections to this requirement as it meant that Ontario would have to launch health insurance reform without knowing whether federal support would be forthcoming (e.g., whether a sufficient number of other provinces would sign on). Moreover, Ontario had serious objections to the universal (i.e., compulsory) nature of the proposed plan. The Ontario position was that it could not make the program compulsory although coverage would be universally available and the government would informally guarantee an initial enrollment of 85 percent of the Ontario population (Taylor 1987, 221). Most simply, in the political calculation of the Ontario government, compulsion implied the need for enforcement, and enforcement raised the specter of public resentment and political recrimination (Taylor 1987, 122). The federal conditions and provincial reaction created a stalemate. Fully one year later, the federal government had not changed its requirements, and only three provinces—which did not include Ontario—had signed on.

Now the federal government was under increasingly serious electoral pressure and felt that it needed to reach an agreement before the impending federal election (Taylor 1987, 222, 223, 225). The Liberal government was in serious political trouble as a result of widespread perceptions of arrogance focused in large part on the Pipeline Debate of 1956.[2] The Progressive Conservative Party was attempting to outflank the Liberal Party on social issues and charged that the federal Liberal Party was bluffing in its offer to provide a federal cost-sharing program for public health insurance (Taylor 1987, 156). In response, the Liberal Party adopted what had become (and would remain) an age-old Liberal political tactic: campaign to the left and govern to the right. With an election imminent, it was now time for the former.

With the Ontario government already publicly committed to health insurance if federal aid was forthcoming, the federal government backed away from its insistence on a universal plan. In doing so, it accepted what, in Ontario, amounted to a voluntary plan (Taylor 1987, 223). The federal government also softened its position on minimum provincial involvement. If the federal government had not concluded agreements with any other province by a specified time, it would consider a separate plan for Ontario only (Taylor 1987, 225). There was little basis on which Ontario might rescind its earlier commitment in the face of the public expectations it had already generated (Taylor 1987, 137). This cleared the way for an agreement in principle between the federal government and Ontario that was sufficient for the federal government to proceed with legislation. Thus, despite the fact that neither the federal government nor the government of Ontario was keen about the prospect of public hospital insurance, the Hospital Insurance and Diagnostic Services Act (HIDS) was passed unanimously by all four parties in the House of Commons in mid-1957 in the face of an upcoming federal election. The Conservative minority government, replacing the Liberals in the 1957 election, removed the six-province requirement, thus cementing the program.

Under HIDS, provincial expenditures for hospital insurance and diagnostic services would be matched by the federal government so long as provinces met various, relatively rigorous conditions.[3] In Taylor's assessment, "It was indeed a tough contract that provinces were required to sign, almost as if the federal government were retaliating for being pushed into a proposal it had not wanted" (Taylor 1990, 93). While provincial plans did not have to be compulsory, they had to be universally available on uniform terms and conditions. That is, public hospital insurance programs could not be means tested or income tested, nor could they subsidize private voluntary plans.

Thus, the health insurance reforms that had failed a decade earlier were partially achieved. Ironically, this took place under the leadership of two governments opposed to public hospital insurance in principle. Moreover, hospital insurance was brought in at a point when it no longer enjoyed CMA support—having failed to pass when it had that support.[4] The dynamics of federal–provincial interaction stood at the center of this apparent paradox.

Explaining the Central Characteristics of the Hospital Insurance Plan

Certain characteristics of the hospital insurance plan as adopted later contributed to the rise of public health insurance to iconic status in Canada. They also helped foster public health insurance's role as a powerful tool of territorial integration. However, it is critical to note that, for the most part, these characteristics were incidental elements of the federal plan.

Certainly the federal program recognized and reinforced a central role for the provinces in shaping their own hospital insurance programs. The program was relatively conditional and certainly more highly conditional than future programs, such as federal cost-sharing for medical care insurance, would be. However, at the same time, it was not nearly as specific in its conditions as the initial federal proposal (based on the Heagerty recommendations) had been in 1943. The sequencing of events was crucial in this outcome. The failure of federal reforms in 1945 had opened up political space for the provinces to proceed on their own, and some of them did. In the wake of provincial experimentation, the federal government simply could not enforce a specific model of hospital insurance on the provinces once four provinces already had programs fully operating (Taylor 1987, 202).

At the same time, the federal conditions on cost-sharing for hospital insurance introduced elements that helped make public health insurance a symbol of national unity and identity—including universality and public insurance as an entitlement unrestricted by payment of premiums or coinsurance fees. Policymakers, however, did not deliberately intend either of these outcomes. Despite later revisionist histories that elevated universality to iconic status as a philosophic principle underpinning the health care system in Canada, the requirement that insurance be universally available on uniform terms and conditions simply meant that federal cost-sharing funds could not be used to subsidize insurance provision through private plans—thus banning the transfer of public funds to private control. This provision reflected a desire to keep direct public control over public funds more than a commitment to egalitarian ideals (Naylor 1986, 166).

A similarly unintended effect took place with regard to coinsurance (user fees) and premiums. The federal government simply wanted to ensure that increases in its own contributions would be directly tied to increases in the provincial financial contribution in order to provide incentives for provincial governments to exercise strong cost control. As a result, expenditures financed by payments from patients were not eligible for federal matching.[5] Thus, the federal matching grant would actually be lower than otherwise would be the case to the degree that hospital insurance costs were financed through coinsurance fees, deductibles, or premiums. Only Alberta and British Columbia (which had already instituted coinsurance payments in 1950) ever imposed such fees, and these were phased out by the mid-1980s. Similarly, these fiscal arrangements had the unanticipated effect of discouraging provincial reliance on premiums. The provinces that had premiums abandoned them, and by 1973 only Ontario continued to enforce hospital insurance premiums (Taylor 1990, 95). Although the federal program did not proscribe premiums or user fees and had not envisioned a system free of these elements, it inadvertently created significant disincentives to rely on such funding mechanisms, and they faded, at least temporarily, from the public health insurance landscape.[6]

The movement away from user fees and premiums, in conjunction with the reinterpretation of universality, transformed these programs from insurance programs into regular benefit programs, at least in terms of their financing structure. Programs structured on an insurance basis are typically thought to be more politically resistant to change or retrenchment because benefits, in contrast, are an earned entitlement. However, in Canada the shift away from the concept of health insurance as earned through the payment of premiums helped set the stage for the growing perception of entitlement to public health insurance on a different basis—as a right of citizenship.

Explaining Divergence in National-level Reforms in the United States and Canada

Influential arguments based on the notion of path dependence have emerged to explain the divergent development of public health insurance in the United States and Canada. Most notably, Jacob Hacker, as outlined above, has argued that the passage of national health insurance faces virtually insurmountable obstacles in countries where private insurance coverage expands before the implementation of public insurance, public insurance plans are initially categorical, and efforts to expand the medical industry take place before access is made universal. The development of public health insurance in Canada challenges this interpretation on all three counts.

Voluntary Health Insurance Coverage

Differences in voluntary health insurance coverage do not provide a compelling explanation of divergent developments in the United States and Canada. Hacker's basic argument is that the broadening coverage of voluntary insurance displaced the need for public coverage and created a set of interests hostile to government intervention in health insurance. Thus differences in levels of voluntary health insurance can help explain why reform was successful in Canada (where coverage rates were lower) and unsuccessful in the United States (where coverage rates were higher).

First, on a number of counts, the data on voluntary insurance coverage do not support this conclusion. The difference in voluntary health insurance coverage in the two countries appears too slim to provide a compelling explanation of the large divergence in outcomes. Hacker compares voluntary health insurance coverage in Canada and the United States in 1957 and finds significant differences between the two countries, with 70 percent coverage in the United States in comparison with 45 percent coverage in Canada (see table 7.1). If, however, one compares coverage in Canada in 1957, when health insurance reform was passed into law, with coverage

Table 7.1   Voluntary Private Health Insurance Coverage, United States (1950 and 1956) and Canada (1956)

	United States		Canada, 1956		Ontario
	1950	1956	Unadjusted	Adjusted	1956
Coverage (of population)	50.5	70.1	44.7	54.3	74.4

Source: Somers and Somers, 1961, 543, 547; National Health and Welfare, 1958, 4–5.

in the United States in 1950, when national health insurance was defeated, the relevant U.S. coverage rate is nearer to 50 percent and much more comparable to Canadian coverage rates.

Furthermore, the coverage rates for Canada used in these comparisons do not take into account the fact that some provinces already had public hospital insurance, thus depressing national levels of voluntary health insurance.[7] In 1956 the coverage rate in Canada (excluding provinces that already had public hospital insurance coverage—that is, Saskatchewan, British Columbia, Alberta, and Newfoundland) was over 54 percent—higher than U.S. coverage rates in 1950 when national health insurance failed. Coverage rates in both Canada and the United States also varied widely on a state/province basis largely as a result of the differing levels of industrialization between primarily urban and primarily rural areas. In Ontario, where the adoption of hospital insurance was critical to the initiation of a federal plan, 74 percent of the population was covered by voluntary hospital insurance in 1956 when hospital insurance reform was successfully undertaken. This figure is higher than the national coverage rate in the United States in 1957 and considerably higher than the roughly 50 percent coverage in the United States in the early 1950s when health insurance reforms failed.

Second, the chronology of the extension of insurance coverage by type of health service in Canada runs contrary to the expectations generated by this strand of path-dependent analysis. Public hospital insurance in Canada emerged earlier and with much less resistance than medical care insurance even though voluntary insurance coverage for hospital services was much more widespread than was voluntary medical care insurance (Taylor 1987, 199). The pattern of difference between these two policy areas suggests a conclusion similar to that suggested by patterns of support for public insurance among American regions as discussed in chapter 4—support for public health insurance was highest in those regions and for service types in which voluntary coverage was highest. The Canadian case illustrates that the political dynamics generated by voluntary health insurance coverage were not preordained. Voluntary private insurance in Canada had the reverse effect to that hypothesized by Hacker—the more successful prepayment plans and private insurance were at demonstrating the advantages of insurance, the greater the public demand to extend coverage to everyone through public programs (Taylor 1990, 66).

The existence of a strong system of private benefits generated highly contradictory dynamics in Ontario. On the one hand, the growth of private benefits had created a set of commercial interests that would be, of course, strongly opposed to universal public hospital benefits. That said, Ontario Premier Leslie Frost did not seem particularly concerned with this opposition and took several opportunities to publicly challenge the industry.[8] While generating oppositional interests, the existence of a well-established set of private benefits in Ontario also simultaneously facilitated the adoption of a system of public benefits.[9]

- The private benefits established public acceptance of the collective insurance principle.
- The system created a ready-made revenue source with the Ontario government viewing private premiums as a preexisting self-imposed tax.
- The extent of private benefits assuaged policymakers' concerns about compliance and achievement of universal coverage. The Ontario government proceeded in the belief that the large portion of the population that was already covered would be moved easily to public coverage.
- Private benefits helped address a critical issue of administrative capacity as the province simply converted the largest nonprofit voluntary insurance Blue Cross plan to become the public agency administering the new public program.

Ironically, had Ontario faced a clean slate in terms of private benefits, as did Saskatchewan, the obstacles to moving ahead on hospital insurance might have been much more difficult to overcome. These obstacles mattered less in Saskatchewan because of its relatively small size and the strong municipal system that was used to collect premiums (Taylor 1987, 119–20).

Third, to the degree that voluntary insurance creates a set of interests hostile to public insurance, the structure for providing private health insurance was generally similar in the two countries. A comparison of the voluntary insurance industry in the two countries in the mid-1950s, which examines the division of the market between commercial and not-for-profit carriers as well as the control of the latter by provider-controlled organizations (as well as the division between hospital association and physician-sponsored plans), concludes that the only significant variation between the two was in the greater relative degree of concentration in Canada.[10] The higher concentration of the industry in Canada made it even more likely that insurance industry would be able to oppose government intervention in the provision of health insurance.

At the same time, sequencing—the expansion of voluntary insurance prior to the advent of public programs—had significant effects on public programs in Canada. The existence of voluntary insurance did not prevent the development of public insurance in Canada, but existing voluntary coverage had important implications for the structure and characteristics of subsequent public programs. In Ontario, for example, the government was clearly aware that there were limits to the degree to which it could challenge procedures regarding benefits and pricing, conditions of entitlement, control mechanisms, and revenue collection already established under the system of voluntary insurance (Taylor 1987, 120). Thus, for example, the existence of a system of premiums for voluntary insurance constituted a ready-made system of revenue for public insurance, and financing decisions by the Ontario government were strongly biased in this direction from the outset (Taylor 1987, 120).

Rather than the argument that differences in coverage rates led to large-scale policy divergence, broad similarities in voluntary insurance coverage in both countries contributed to the similar characteristics of public insurance programs as they developed in each country. In both countries, voluntary health insurance contributed to the embeddedness of two central elements of the existing health services system—private physician practice and fee-for-service remuneration. In both systems, public insurance (whether universal or categorical) did not challenge these two central elements of the existing system. This implies a very different mechanism of sequencing and lock-in than outlined in existing path-dependent explanations.

Existence of Categorical Programs and Efforts to Expand the Medical Industry

The evidence from the Canadian case does not support the contention that the existence of categorical programs undermines the subsequent development of universal programs. Prior to the federal proposal for comprehensive health insurance in 1945, all provinces provided for "grants to hospitals and for the hospitalization of indigent patients" (Grauer 1939, 47). Categorical health insurance programs existed in five of the ten provinces at the time that the federal hospital insurance program became a reality. Comprehensive categorical health insurance programs existed in both Saskatchewan and British Columbia prior to the advent of universal hospital insurance programs in those provinces. In Ontario, which as argued above was key to the inception of a federal hospital insurance program, a program of physician insurance for social assistance recipients, old-age security recipients, and blind pension recipients had existed since the mid-1930s. Rather than undermining political support for universal programs, the effects of these categorical programs conform more closely to the expectations of policymakers in the Medicare era in the United States that categorical programs would spur demand for universal programs. As argued in chapter 5, the reason they did not do so in the U.S. context was a result of the particular characteristics and timing of the Medicare and Medicaid programs rather than path dependence resulting from their categorical program structure.

Neither does the Canadian case support the claim that the buildup of the medical industry before the universalization of access created a serious barrier to public health insurance reform. Efforts to build up the medical industry occurred at the same time in the United States and Canada, and this buildup had proceeded to roughly the same degree in the two countries. Federal grants for hospital construction, similar to those in operation in the United States under Hill–Burton, had been in operation in Canada for roughly a decade at the time national hospital insurance was implemented. As Tuohy notes, "The impact of the federal hospital grants programs on the hospital sector, moreover, was similar in the two countries. In each, the for-profit hospital sector, always small, declined further in significance" (1999, 47). In the Canadian example there is no evidence that such grants undermined public programs of universal insurance, and according to Prime Minister Mackenzie King, the grants at the time were thought to represent "the first stages in the development of a comprehensive health insurance plan for all Canada" (Taylor 1990, 81).

Rather than preventing public health program development, the existence of voluntary programs and buildup of the medical industry prior to the advent of public programs shaped the central characteristics of subsequent public programs in both countries. These similar sequences of development in the United States and Canada help to explain a number of the similarities in the contemporary health care systems in the two countries rather than differences between them.

Extending Coverage by Service Area

It is not surprising that in the wake of the failure of more-comprehensive reform, Canadian federal reform proceeded by extending coverage to particular categories of service (such as hospital care, medical care) rather than by category of recipient. First, Saskatchewan already had a program of hospital reform, making this the most logical area in which to extend cost-sharing as well as making cost-sharing for services provided to a particular category of recipients difficult as this would cut against the grain of existing programs. Second, there was no strong precedent (such as Social Security in the United States) for categorical provision. Third, the categorical approach in the United States was initially adopted for very particular reasons— that the program would reprise the compromises of the New Deal and exclude much of the southern African American labor force. Just as had been the case in California earlier, when comprehensive reform failed, reform efforts turned to extending public health insurance by area of service provision.

Conclusions about Expanding Coverage

The history of public health insurance reform in Canada in this period highlights the tenuous nature of this reform. The implementation of hospital insurance in Canada was not the automatic or necessary result either of political culture or the configuration of political institutions nor did it flow naturally from earlier provincial reforms. At various points, relatively slight changes in circumstances might well have led to significantly different outcomes. For example, had the particular alignment of electoral cycles in Ontario and at the federal level not occurred, it is unlikely that a sufficiently strong dynamic auguring in favor of a federal–provincial hospital insurance program would have emerged. Had the federal Liberals not been replaced by the Conservative government in 1957 with its orientation toward federal–provincial reconciliation, the federal government might have held fast to its six-province minimum for cost-sharing for hospital insurance and refused to implement the plan.

The advent of a federal–provincial plan proved momentous. Provinces such as Saskatchewan and British Columbia, which were already providing hospital insurance, were now reimbursed for roughly half their costs—a considerable windfall. In the absence of a federal contribution, Saskatchewan simply could not have afforded to move forward with expansions to its system of public health insurance. With federal contributions for hospital insurance relieving it of a considerable portion of the financial burden, the Saskatchewan provincial government was able to move forward with medical care insurance.

Medical Care Insurance in Saskatchewan

The advent of federal cost-sharing for hospital insurance allowed the provincial government in Saskatchewan the financial latitude to move ahead with medical care insurance. In stark contrast with the earlier development of hospital insurance in Saskatchewan, the decision to embark on public medical care insurance was made with no expectation that federal cost-sharing would be forthcoming and was truly a decision to "go it alone." There were, of course, strong precedents on which to base the expansion of health insurance to the coverage of physician services in Saskatchewan, including the hospital insurance scheme that had in been in operation for roughly fifteen years as well as the more geographically limited experiment in comprehensive coverage in the Swift Current Region. Nevertheless, from the outset the success of this venture was far from assured. Despite contemporary claims that Saskatchewan had a political culture strongly predisposed toward public medical insurance, the endeavor encountered serious resistance from the medical profession, broad segments of the public, and the media. Despite this opposition, universal medical care insurance became a reality—but only after a bitter twenty-three-day physician strike that made news around the world.

The Uncertainty of Reform

The main source of opposition to the provincial plan was the medical profession. Its strength, relative to that of the Saskatchewan government, was at least equal to—if not greater than—the strength of the AMA relative to the U.S. federal government and state medical societies relative to their state governments. Moreover, it was no more predisposed toward public medical insurance than its American counterparts.

The organizational structure of the medical profession in Saskatchewan gave it political advantages not enjoyed in many other Canadian provinces or by physician associations in the United States, including the AMA. As was the case in British Columbia and Alberta, the Saskatchewan College of Physicians and Surgeons (which exercised public authority to regulate the profession especially in regard to licensing) and the provincial medical association (representing the interests of doctors) were combined (Naylor 1986, 96; see also Taylor 1990, 98–99). As a result, membership in the professional association was required and individual doctors could not register dissent with association policies by resigning their membership from the professional association without giving up their license to practice. Furthermore, the college controlled the two major (and expanding) prepayment plans for physician services in the province and, thus, had sole control over the policies governing voluntary insurance, including enrollment, benefits, methods, and amounts of payment (Taylor 1990, 99). This translated into significant economic and political power for the college.

Given this power, as Taylor compellingly argues, the college could be viewed as being tantamount to a private government in the heath care field: "One could say that in Saskatchewan there were two governments in the field of health, a private and a public one, each with its own legislature, cabinet, bureaucracy, revenue system, territorial domain, and political ideology. Any action by one to encroach on the territory of the other was to invite certain conflict" (Taylor 1990, 99–100). For example, the development of profession-controlled plans had "irrevocably institutionalized" the fee-for-service payment method, and any attempt to implement a different payment method was believed to be futile (Taylor 1987, 268).

The doctors had already experienced some success in forestalling earlier attempts at expansion of public insurance coverage for physician services at the regional level. In 1955 proposals for two additional comprehensive regional medical care plans (following the model of the Swift Current plan) were subject to referendums in their respective areas. The college and its voluntary prepayment plans launched a massive publicity campaign contributing to the resounding defeat of medical care in both regions (Taylor 1990, 98; Naylor 1986, 179). These earlier battles had contributed to reinforcing the solidarity of the profession as well as steeling their resolve to resist further expansions of public medical care insurance (Taylor 1990, 98).

The doctors had also aggressively adopted a strategy of expanding physician-controlled voluntary prepayment plans (Taylor 1990, 98). Roughly 40 percent of the population was already covered under enrollment in the two profession-sponsored plans (Naylor 1986, 179; Taylor 1987, 266n71). Furthermore, the province also had a categorical system of comprehensive coverage for recipients of old-age pensions and social assistance for more than sixteen years at the time when universal medical care insurance became a reality. Thus roughly one-quarter of the Saskatchewan population had "more or less" comprehensive coverage for medical services under various public programs including the Swift Current plan for comprehensive health service coverage in that region, the social assistance medical care program, and the municipal doctor contract system (Naylor 1986, 177). Only the remaining one-third of the population was without medical care coverage.

In addition to its own considerable political power, the College of Physicians and Surgeons received the support of extraprovincial interests including the CMA and the insurance industry, which were both committed to defeating public physician service insurance in Saskatchewan. This support significantly increased the pressure the college could bring to bear on the provincial government (Taylor 1990, 105). The Saskatchewan government was confronted not only by its own physicians but also by the national profession.

The financial resources at the disposal of the college were, in proportional terms, substantial. Using ballpark comparisons, the doctors in Saskatchewan spent somewhere between two and a half to over three and a half times the amount per capita as the oft-noted publicity campaigns by the medical profession against public health insurance in the United States. For the 1960 election, the college assessed its members $100 for funds to wage a campaign against the CCF (Taylor 1990, 104). In conjunction with funds from the CMA, the college spent $100,000 in the 1960 Saskatchewan provincial election—roughly $110 per 1,000 population (Naylor 1986, 185). By comparison, the entire California Medical Association campaign against public health insurance in California in 1945 was estimated at roughly $250,000 (Harris 1966, 33), or approximately $35 per 1,000 population in 1965 dollars. In 1948 AMA members were assessed $25 (voluntarily paid in the first year by two-thirds of the membership—the same proportion as paid the $100 assessment in Saskatchewan in 1960) to amass a war chest of $3.5 million (Harris, 1966, 39–40), or approximately $30 per 1,000 population in 1965 dollars. In the 1964 battle against Medicare, it was rumored that the AMA intended to spend up to $8 million in conjunction with state medical societies (Harris 1966, 182), or roughly $40 per 1,000 population.

Finally, the coalition of interests opposed to the Saskatchewan plan was as broad as the coalition resisting public insurance in the United States. In the 1960 provincial election the college was joined in its opposition to public medical care insurance by the Saskatchewan Liberal Party, the dental and pharmaceutical associations, and the Chambers of Commerce (Taylor 1990, 104). During the actual doctors' strike in 1962, the press was universally critical (Taylor 1990, 118–19). Popular resistance to medical care insurance was organized through the development of a series of Keep Our Doctors Committees, which were vocally and vociferously opposed to the plan. These committees staged a series of impressive public rallies against the medical insurance plan.

The anti-insurance coalition also used rhetoric as drastic and misleading as the AMA campaigns in the United States. As noted by Lord Taylor, a leading figure in resolving the Saskatchewan doctors' strike, "The American Medical Association was at this time, hysterically opposed to Medicare; and it endeavored, not without some success, to communicate its hysteria to the doctors and the public in Saskatchewan" (quoted in Taylor 1990, 121). Organized medicine in Saskatchewan portrayed public health insurance as communistic and a threat to freedom. Typical press coverage in Saskatchewan referred to the medical insurance program as "ferocious" and the government as "dedicated to the destruction of our economic system" (Taylor 1990, 118–19).

The 1962 Doctors' Strike and Its Resolution

In response to the announcement of Premier Douglas during a provincial by-election campaign in early 1959 that the provincial government intended "to embark upon a comprehensive medical care program that would cover all our people," the college emphasized its support for voluntary prepayment plans that, in this case, it controlled.[11] To the degree the college was willing to countenance a role for government in health insurance, it argued in favor of the CMA policy of subsidizing coverage for low-income people provided through voluntary agencies (Taylor 1990, 106). As outlined above, the college waged a massive publicity campaign in the 1960 election.

Initially the CCF government was far from certain as to how the public would react to the plan (Taylor 1987, 269). In the 1960 election the government received only 40 percent of the vote. In reaction to these results, "the college contended that the election, which had been virtually converted into a referendum on medical care insurance, had indicated majority opposition to the government's policy" (Taylor 1990, 104). In the 1962 federal election the CCF was badly beaten in Saskatchewan (including the defeat of former CCF premier Tommy Douglas who had left provincial politics to run federally), and this defeat was widely perceived to be a reaction against public medical care insurance (Taylor 1987, 300). Nevertheless, an internal assessment presented by the head of the college to the CMA in July 1962 noted: "Over the past two and a half years, the public in that province seems to have accepted and approved of the fact that they will be provided with some form of plan for comprehensive, all-inclusive medical care insurance" (Taylor 1990, 114). Rather than responding to public opinion demanding public insurance, the CCF was shaping public opinion.

Despite the strident opposition of the profession, legislation was introduced and passed in the fall of 1961 making provision for a compulsory, premium-based system of public medical insurance. In response, the primary objective of the college was to preserve a role for the prepayment plans in the expectation that the CCF government would be replaced after the next election. If the move to public insurance was to later be reversed, the college believed it was critical that the prepayment plans survive so they might provide a voluntary alternative to the public program (Taylor 1990, 116). In response to the college's refusal to even negotiate in regards to a public plan, the government offered a major concession: The doctors could directly bill their patients who would then be reimbursed by the public plan according to the negotiated fee schedule. The college rejected the concession and called again for a system of subsidization of voluntary plans (Taylor 1990, 109). The gulf between the two sides could not be bridged, and on July 1, 1962, the doctors withdrew their services.

The strike presented huge political risks for both sides—no one knew where the public would lay blame if deaths were attributed to the strike (Taylor 1987, 314). Under mounting pressure, after twenty-three days an agreement was reached as a result of a major concession on both sides. The medical profession agreed to accept that the plan would be universal and compulsory with the government collecting premiums and disbursing payments. For its part, the government agreed that the existing organizational structure of the voluntary plans remain in place to act as billing and payment agents for physicians who did not wish to deal directly with the government health commission (Taylor 1990, 125).[12]

With the strike ended, universal compulsory public health insurance for physician services was fully in operation in the province of Saskatchewan although the physician-controlled prepayment plan organizations remained in place. The medical profession viewed the end of the strike as a cease-fire rather than a cessation of hostilities (Taylor 1987, 325–27). As the profession's leadership had hoped, twenty-one months later, in early 1964, the CCF government fell and the Liberals, who had opposed the public medical insurance plan and supported the doctors, were elected. But "to the surprise of many of the public and the dismay of the profession, the

Liberal government did not change the format of the program, and the profession-controlled plans were never returned to their prior status" (Taylor 1990, 129). Comprehensive universal compulsory health insurance in Saskatchewan had become a reality.

Conclusions

The development of public hospital insurance in this period presents a contrasting perspective to path-dependent interpretations of developments in the United States. The development of categorical programs for health insurance, efforts to expand voluntary insurance coverage, and efforts to expand the medical industry prior to the universalization of access—all of the factors argued to explain the failure of national health insurance in the United States—were present but did not prevent the advent of universal hospital insurance in Canada. Successful reform in Canada undermines the argument that this set of factors necessitated the failure of public health insurance in the United States.

Rather than relatively limited differences in private insurance coverage explaining the major divergence in the development of public programs in the United States and Canada, the similarities in voluntary coverage in both countries powerfully explain the similarities in the public programs that emerged—the predominance of fee-for-service remuneration under public programs and the entrenching of private medical practice. Neither of these two elements of health provision was seriously open to question in either country following the expansion of voluntary insurance in each.

At the same time, while the factors outlined above did not necessitate the failure to develop universal public insurance in Canada, the development of a national program for universal hospital insurance in Canada was highly contingent and, in retrospect, seems much more fortuitous than path dependent. Successful provincial hospital insurance reforms did not automatically translate into federal reform in Canada, and the Canadian example provides little reason to expect, following Mitchell's argument outlined in chapter 2, that successful state health insurance programs would have likely done so in the United States. In the case of hospital insurance, however, federal–provincial dynamics contributed to the adoption of a national program of universal hospital insurance. Even more powerful dynamics generated by the politics of territorial integration soon emerged and pushed Canada even further in its own distinctive direction of development.

CHAPTER EIGHT

Medical Care Insurance in Canada, 1962–84

I suppose we'll be proposing grocery-care next.

Ernest Manning, Premier of Alberta

The principles of the Canada Health Act began as simple conditions attached to federal funding for medicare. Over time, they became much more than that. Today, they represent . . . the values underlying the health care system. . . . The principles have stood the test of time and continue to reflect the values of Canadians.

Roy J. Romanow, Health Canada Act Overview

I T IS DIFFICULT TO OVERSTATE the seriousness of the crisis facing Canadian unity during the period in which medical care insurance was debated and introduced. As *independentiste* sentiment in Québec flared, bombings first took place in Québec's largest city, Montréal, in 1963. The tension reached crisis proportions seven years later when, in the wake of the kidnapping of the British Trade Commissioner James Cross and kidnapping and murder of Québec cabinet minister Pierre Laporte, the federal government temporarily suspended civil liberties across Canada on the basis of "apprehended insurrection" in Québec. Over this period, the rise of the militant separatist movement, the Front de Liberation du Québec (FLQ), as well as the creation of nonviolent parties dedicated to the establishment of an independent Québec by constitutional means—such as the Rassemblement pour l'Indépendence Nationale in 1960 and Ralliement National in 1966, which were both superseded by the Parti Québécois (PQ) in 1968—signaled the force of this challenge to Canada's territorial integrity.[1] It was from within this context that a national system of medical care insurance emerged in Canada.

Medicare, in common Canadian usage, is generally used to refer to both hospital insurance and medical care insurance. In the United States, common usage is more precise and refers to public insurance for seniors. To avoid confusion, the term *Medicare* will be used to refer to the U.S. program. In discussing insurance provided under the rubric of the Medicare Act (1966) in Canada, I will refer to *medical care* or *physician care insurance.*

The development of national public medical care insurance in Canada is often viewed as the result of a relatively natural evolution flowing out of earlier federal and provincial policy innovations such as universal hospital care insurance at the federal level and medical care insurance in Saskatchewan. The development and consolidation of national universal medical care insurance, however, in the period from the mid-1960s to the mid-1980s was highly tenuous. In this contingent process of development, the conjuncture at key points between the politics of health care and politics of territorial integration played an important role. Powerful political currents—especially those developing in Québec—provided a central dynamic driving the development of a national system of medical care insurance designed to touch the lives of all Canadians regardless of where they lived.

The Introduction of a Federal Program for Medical Care Insurance in Canada, 1960–71

Following the advent of provincial reforms in Saskatchewan, the political conditions were not very favorable to the development of a federal program of public physician-care insurance. Nevertheless, the politics of territorial integration—especially the perception on the part of federal policymakers that public medical care insurance could be used as a powerful tool of territorial integration—provided an important dynamic driving reform.

National Medical Care Insurance as a Linear Progression

The argument has been made that provincial innovations in public health insurance were central to federal reforms. Hacker argues that "the provinces proved to be a crucial incubator of policy activism" and "provincial efforts later paved the way for national legislation" (1998, 72). Tuohy also emphasizes the degree to which federal legislation is seen to have flowed out of provincial innovations, arguing that the major difference between the development of public health insurance in Canada and the United States was policy innovation at the provincial level: "The two countries differed in one important respect. Whereas Canadian provincial governments became the loci of experimentation with governmental hospital insurance, American state governments did not" (1999, 47).

Provincial reforms are argued to have contributed to federal reform in a number of ways. First, they acted as "demonstration projects" both for other provinces and federal policymakers (Hacker 1998, 96). Tuohy carefully points out that medical care insurance in Saskatchewan had both negative and positive demonstration effects; however, in her analysis, the degree to which the Saskatchewan program demonstrated the feasibility of universal public medical care insurance outweighed the former (Tuohy 1999, 53). In addition, these innovations are argued to have "served as test cases that defused conflict with opponents of the reformers, particularly doctors" (Maioni 1998, 160). Finally, they are argued to have encouraged provincial leaders to demand federal funding for provincially provided programs (Hacker 1998, 96).

A second line of reasoning that ties the development of public medical care insurance back to earlier policy development is the argument that the federal program of hospital insurance created the expectation that medical care insurance would naturally follow. Medical care insurance "had become a natural, normal expectation" that awaited only the right time for implementation (Taylor 1990, 143). In a similar vein, Maioni argues that the development of medical care insurance represented the "consolidation of existing federal–provincial arrangements based on universal health insurance principles. The debate centered not on providing health insurance to certain groups [as in the United States] but on the extension of benefits beyond hospital insurance to cover the costs of medical care" (Maioni 1998, 119). In turn, as argued above, the development of federal hospital care insurance is also often viewed as the logical extension of provincial hospital care insurance schemes—especially that of Saskatchewan, which had been developed more than a decade earlier. Thus the evolution of the contemporary Canadian system is seen as unfolding from this single point of departure—the advent of universal public hospital insurance in Saskatchewan in 1947.

Electoral considerations are typically central in these explanations of federal action on the medical care insurance front. The Liberals faced an emerging threat from the left by the New Democratic Party (NDP) that, having been formed out of the CCF in 1962 and having Tommy Douglas as its leader, could claim the adoption of medical care insurance in Saskatchewan as its own. As a result, the governing Liberals faced pressure in the House of Commons from the NDP to develop a national health insurance system based on the Saskatchewan model (Maioni 1998, 130; Hacker 1998, 103, 104).[2] The NDP had made medicare the central plank of its election platform in both 1962 and 1963. In response, public insurance for medical care was a central plank in the Liberal platforms of 1962, 1963, and 1965 (Gordon 1977, 224; La Marsh 1969, 122; Newman 1968, 412). Following the election of 1965, it is argued that the governing Liberals then felt compelled to introduce the program in light of these electoral commitments or, alternatively, were forced to do so by virtue of their need to maintain the support of the NDP.[3] Underpinning this line of reasoning is a broader argument regarding the key role of the configuration of Canadian political institutions in encouraging the development of third parties at the provincial level, which, in turn, contributed to the development of the NDP as a powerful electoral force at the national level.

The arguments that focus on earlier developments at the provincial level typically tie the development of public medical care insurance in Canada back to the configuration of political institutions. For example, because federal innovations followed from provincial innovations, the central question becomes "why and how did the provinces take the lead in enacting first hospital insurance and then comprehensive medical insurance?" (Hacker 1998, 100). The answer to this question, for Hacker, is institutional. First, federalism created opportunities for provincial parties supportive of reform to gain power, and as a result, "Canadian federalism fostered the development of provincial programs that could serve as examples to neighbouring provinces and eventually form the basis for national legislation" (Hacker 1998, 99).

Second, federal grants equalized the fiscal capacity of provinces, provided the prospect that federal transfers would become available for health programs, and, in provinces that already had eligible programs as cost-sharing became available, freed up funds for further policy entrepreneurship (Hacker 1998, 101).[4] Underpinning these explanations is a focus on political institutions and, especially, the impacts of Canadian federalism. As argued below, however, the dynamics driving federal reform were rooted in the linguistic tensions inherent in Canadian society and the associated political tumult.

Political Resistance to Federal Medical Care Insurance

While it is often argued that the development of public medical care insurance in Saskatchewan set in motion positive feedback dynamics that created pressure for federal reforms, the political context for federal medical care insurance proposals in the wake of the developments in Saskatchewan was not particularly propitious. Although universal public medical care insurance had been implemented in Saskatchewan, this development, in itself, triggered negative feedback dynamics auguring against the adoption of a similar program at the federal level. First, it generated even more serious resistance by the CMA to public physician-care insurance at the national level than had existed prior to the Saskatchewan experiment. Second, it contributed to the adoption of alternative health insurance plans in other provinces. Finally, it created serious concern at the federal level about the degree of resistance that a federal program might encounter.

One of the crucial effects of Saskatchewan adopting medical services insurance was to steel the CMA's resolve against compulsory public insurance for physician services. Organized medicine in Canada viewed the development of public medical care insurance in Saskatchewan as a "serious breach" (Taylor 1990, 129). In response to the developments in Saskatchewan, the president of the CMA made a "ringing call to the profession to reinforce the private governmental structure it had created to prevent any further breach in the system. And it made very clear its fear of, and determination to exclude, any other influence in the arrangements the profession controlled" (Taylor 1990, 130). As the CMA campaigned vigorously against national medical insurance, it issued constant warnings that "the introduction of medical care insurance, which they pejoratively referred to as socialized medicine, would lead to an exodus of doctors from the country" (Taylor 1990, 26).

Furthermore, in the wake of Saskatchewan's adoption of medicare, Alberta, Ontario, and British Columbia began introducing programs designed to reinforce voluntary insurance and physician-controlled prepayment programs—a major breakthrough for the CMA and the Canadian Health Insurance Association (CHIA) (Taylor 1990, 133). This interpretation contrasts sharply with that of Hacker, who argues that "provincial governments in British Columbia, Alberta and Ontario moved almost immediately to consider plans that followed the Saskatchewan precedent" (1998, 100). Hacker's assertion that the British Columbia, Alberta, and Ontario plans were highly consistent with the Saskatchewan plan is a key element in his argument that federal reform was the result of a relatively linear progression stemming from adoption of medical care insurance in Saskatchewan. These plans, however, were clearly intended as *alternatives* to the Saskatchewan plan.

Proposals in Alberta went furthest in this regard. Alberta passed legislation for income-based subsidization of private insurance coverage in early 1963. The program was a direct response to the adoption of public health insurance in Saskatchewan, and the Alberta premier, Ernest Manning, believed that the new program "would give Canadians a program they could set alongside 'the socialistic type of program' in Saskatchewan" (Taylor 1990, 133). Indicative of the philosophical predisposition of the Alberta government, in his testimony to the Hall Commission, the Alberta minister of health stated unequivocally that "his government was opposed to any program of state medical care 'which removes all direct individual financial responsibility; so-called socialized health and medical services are incompatible with the rights and responsibilities inherent in a free and democratic society'" (Taylor 1987, 338). The Alberta program became the prototype for proponents of an alternative to universal compulsory public insurance and had the strong support of the CMA and CHIA, which believed this program needed to succeed in order to stem popular demand for universal public insurance based on the Saskatchewan model.

Other alternatives to universal public insurance coverage were developing in Ontario and British Columbia. Both provinces took a different tack from the Alberta plan by directly providing individual insurance that was subsidized on an income-tested basis while leaving group insurance to the private insurance carriers (Taylor 1990, 134).[5] Despite the differences between the Alberta approach (subsidization of privately provided insurance for low-income persons) and the Ontario/BC approach (government provision of individual insurance, subsidized for low-income persons), none of these three provincial initiatives was propitious for further development of universal public physician care in Canada: "Three of Canada's most powerful provinces had now acted in such a way as to leave the majority of the population who could afford voluntary insurance to the private sector, while governments paid part or all of the costs for the 'poor risks'" (Taylor 1990, 134).

Québec also fell into line with these other provinces before the federal medicare program came into effect. The provincial Liberals appeared to be considering more ambitious plans for medical care insurance reform; however, they were defeated in 1966 by the more conservative Union Nationale, and the policy position of the Québec government shifted to support only for subsidizing health insurance for low-income individuals. Thus the four largest Canadian provinces were committed to public plans that provided or subsidized physician care insurance to those with low incomes while leaving the rest of the population to voluntary insurance for physician care.

The development of these alternative proposals demonstrates the degree to which universal public insurance care was not assumed to be the necessary complement to or natural extension of universal hospital insurance. Certainly the governments of the four largest provinces in Canada did not see this as necessary, natural, or even desirable and had posed a credible alternative. In fact, at points, there appeared to be hints that reinforcing voluntary programs and subsidizing coverage for low-income people was under consideration by the federal government itself. Writing to the cabinet to solicit input on the Throne Speech for 1965, Prime Minister Pearson noted: "I do not think we can plan to take that [medical care insurance] on, at least in any comprehensive way in 1965. But we do need to make some plans for dealing with the greatest needs in this area" (Taylor 1987, 363).

Finally, the Saskatchewan experience generated considerable concern among federal policymakers. The difficulty of implementing medical care insurance in Saskatchewan demonstrated just how politically risky the venture would be for a minority Liberal government at the federal level. Certainly, the Saskatchewan doctors' strike removed any perception at the federal level that medical care insurance would be a natural evolution from hospital care insurance.[6] Federal policymakers were acutely aware that there was "a hell of a lot of opposition" to the plan in Saskatchewan. In light of the developments in Saskatchewan, the federal decision to proceed would have to be made on the assumption that an expansion of public health insurance would be campaigned against vigorously—which it was, especially by the insurance industry, which argued that the federal proposals would "ruin the nation."[7]

The omens for the successful achievement of a national plan "now were increasingly dark" (Taylor 1990, 144). In the view of the CMA, "the odds in favor of the market-economy approach . . . were shifting most favorably" (Taylor 1990, 140). Encouraged by these outcomes, the CMA was stepping up its publicity campaign against universal compulsory public health insurance as well as directly lobbying at the highest political levels.[8] Furthermore, public support of compulsory public physician-care insurance was weak. In a public opinion poll conducted in the fall of 1965 as the government was preparing to introduce legislation, support for a voluntary plan (52 percent) outstripped support for a compulsory plan (41 percent) by a significant margin.[9]

The provinces, on the whole, were recalcitrant. At the annual Provincial Premiers Conference, "so strident were the tones, so angry the voices, and so vehement the opposition that one journalist summed up, 'The federal government's proposed legislation lies torn, tattered, and politically rejected'" (Taylor 1990, 149). When the federal government announced its medical care insurance proposals in 1965, Premier of Alberta Ernest Manning commented acerbically, "I suppose we'll be proposing grocery-care next."[10]

Nevertheless, the Liberal minority government elected in 1963 and reelected as a minority again in 1965 persevered in pursuing a national plan, and the federal government eventually pushed through a conditional cost-sharing program for public medical care insurance. Of course various compromises were made. For example, the medicare program would have "principles" rather than "conditions," a semantic measure intended to make the plan more palatable to the provinces. These principles, later to become enshrined in the CHA, were portability, public administration, comprehensiveness, universality, and accessibility.[11]

From the outset the Québec government flatly refused to participate in any federal scheme in an arena of primarily provincial jurisdiction. Premier of Québec Jean Lésage argued that Québec would bring in its own plan of medical care insurance but that "when our plan is introduced, it will be operated outside any joint Federal–Provincial program in line with our general policy of opting out of all areas within our competence" (quoted in Taylor 1990, 147).[12] The Québec position had been and remained clear: its overriding objectives were complete provincial autonomy in all areas of provincial jurisdiction and securing the financial capacity to fund programs in these areas independently of conditional federal transfers.

This provincial recalcitrance was overcome, however, by a brilliant federal maneuver of dubious constitutional legitimacy—certainly breaking the spirit, if not the letter, of the Canadian constitution. In the fall of 1968 the federal finance minister announced an increase of 2 percent in federal income tax. Although it was formally called the social development tax (as it would have been unconstitutional for the federal government to levy a health care tax), the tax was clearly intended to finance federal contributions to health insurance. Taxpayers in all provinces would be, in essence, paying for medical care insurance regardless of whether or not their province had a program eligible for federal cost-sharing. This action created significant political pressure on provincial governments to acquiesce to the program (Taylor 1987, 392). As a result, all provinces, even those that were less than enthusiastic about the federal plan, such as Québec, quickly developed programs eligible for federal cost-sharing (see table 8.1).

The Politics of Territorial Integration and the Politics of Public Health Insurance

The context from which medical care insurance emerged was marked by powerful tensions between the nation-building aspirations of the federal government and the government in Québec. The clash between these different visions had been ongoing, with many specific issues being resolved in favor of the latter. Québec had first challenged federal conditional grants in 1960. The Liberal Party, while in parliamentary opposition, had adopted a policy in favor of allowing provincial "opting out" from established programs with compensation. After the Liberals returned to power in 1963 as a minority government, the change was agreed to at a federal conference, and Ottawa had also acknowledged the right of provinces to "contract out" of existing shared-cost programs receiving compensation for well-established joint

Table 8.1   Provincial Adoption of Medicare-Eligible Physician-Care Insurance, Canada

Province	Date
Saskatchewan, British Columbia	1968
Newfoundland, Nova Scotia,	
Manitoba, Alberta, Ontario	1969
Quebec, PEI	1970
New Brunswick	1971

Source: Taylor 1990, 149.

programs through tax abatement rather than federal cash transfers. This decision marked a significant change as tax abatements differ significantly from cash transfers in that the only way for the federal government to reclaim tax room ceded to a province is to raise its own tax rates—a move that is highly politically unpopular. The effect of tax abatements is to make transfers essentially unconditional and permanent.

By the mid-1960s, the Province of Québec had already opted out of federal post-secondary education funding (receiving an abatement of corporate taxes in lieu of direct grants to universities), forgone benefits to its citizens under the Unemployment Insurance program, indicated that it would be opting out of federal–provincial cost-sharing for hospital insurance, and was in the midst of constructing its own pension system, the Québec Pension Plan (QPP)—parallel to, but distinct from, the Canadian Pension Plan (CPP).

To varying degrees, some instances of Québec's exercise of provincial autonomy were largely symbolic. For example, Québec had promised not to alter existing services provided under federal–provincial cost-sharing arrangements from which it proposed to opt out. However, in politics—especially territorial, nationalist, and linguistic politics—symbolism is key.[13] Liberal ministers began to feel the pressure of this situation. As Judy La Marsh, minister of health and welfare, noted: "The public felt that we should heed no more of Québec's repeated attacks upon the citadel of a strong federal government." La Marsh and other ministers felt the situation in regard to Québec was increasingly "insupportable" (La Marsh 1969, 123).

Given this context, it was clear that public medical care insurance was not a policy arena that the federal government would willingly cede.

These "national objectives" of Quebec ran counter to four federal government objectives: (1) The necessity of maintaining a direct federal "presence" with Canadian citizens, which could not be limited simply to imposing federal taxes to subsidize provincially-administered programs for which provincial governments presumably received the political credit; (2) The desirability—indeed, in Ottawa's view, the necessity—of maintaining national standards and portability of program rights even in programs such as hospital insurance in which a "contracting out" privilege might be granted after the program had been in operation for some time; (3) The retention of strategic fiscal control of the economy, an objective that would be weakened by outright transfer to the provinces of large spending programs and their accompanying income tax "points"; (4) And, finally, as a Liberal government—fulfillment of a commitment made by the party in 1919 and constantly reiterated thereafter to develop a program of *national* health insurance. (Taylor 1987, 381)

In a context in which provinces could opt out of established programs, a new cost-sharing program offered unique opportunities for renewing a strong federal role. Constitutional questions aside, the relevant political question was whether public opinion in favor of universal medical care insurance was sufficiently strong in Québec that the federal government could put pressure on the provincial government that it could not resist. Federal policymakers were well aware that universal public medical care insurance had as much popular appeal within Québec as anywhere else.[14]

The issue of territorial integration was among the top priorities of the cabinet in this period. Certainly, as Maioni notes, "the Prime Minister considered social programs part of a strategy to strengthen the presence of the federal government and encourage 'nation' building across Canada" (1998, 132). Viewing social programs as instruments of nation-building was, in the words of Tom Kent, former principal assistant to Prime Minister Pearson and the key architect of Canadian social policy at the time, "a perfect expression of the spirit in which we saw things." In the view of federal policymakers, the problem of the Canadian federation was not vertical fiscal imbalance but political imbalance by which the most important functions of government, in the eyes of Canadian citizens, are matters of provincial jurisdiction.[15] As Kent argues, policymakers felt it imperative that "Canada had to become a social union as well as an economic union."[16]

Although there was dissent within the party, this point of view was very powerful in shaping the program on which the Pearson government came to office—reflecting the outlook of both Prime Minister Pearson and his advisers as well as the grassroots of the Liberal Party. The main overarching concern of the Liberal government upon its election in 1963 was "positive Canadianism," which included an emphasis on cooperative federalism. Additional broad concerns were the economy and social policy including, most notably, pensions and medical care insurance.

The initial proposals considered at this time were for a straight federal program for medical care insurance. In an effort to revitalize thinking among small-*l* liberals in Canada, a conference had been held in Kingston, Ontario, in 1960. Tom Kent prepared the main policy paper, and the top priority in Kent's paper was medical care insurance. The recommendations of the Kingston conference worked themselves into policy resolutions presented to a Liberal party rally in January 1961. Medical care insurance became the most important issue of that meeting with the party passing a resolution in favor of the extension of medical care insurance according to a bold plan reminiscent of the original proposals in 1942—the federal government would pay medical care costs for individuals directly.[17] A central rationale for this style of program was that "the glue of Canada needed to be improved by nationwide social policy."[18] In response to constraints on a straight federal approach, Kent himself would, on the election of the Liberals, begin promoting a more limited program that he referred to as Kiddie Care, which proposed a straight federal program of universal health insurance for children—similar to the plan under consideration by the Kennedy administration.[19]

The political prospects for a straight federal program of either a universal or categorical (e.g., limited to children) variety were radically transformed by a number of factors. The first was the report of the Royal Commission on Health Services (Hall Commission) in 1964. The Hall Commission provided, in large part, the philosophical rationale for the expansion of universal public insurance to medical care.[20] The Hall Commission, reflecting its own concern with issues of territorial integration, recommended a "Health Charter," the essence of which was as follows: "The achievement of the highest possible health standards for all our people must become a primary objective of national policy and a cohesive factor contributing to national unity. . . . The objective can best be achieved through a comprehensive, universal Health Services Program for the Canadian people" (Taylor 1990, 135).[21]

The central recommendation of the report, however, was to achieve this coverage through a system of federal–provincial cost-sharing. The rationale was that it was imperative to have all programs for personal health services lodged at the same level of government in order that they be integrated. For federal policymakers, this recommendation made "the politics of a federal plan much more difficult." The Hall Commission was widely seen as having considerable legitimacy, not the least of which was that, having been appointed by a Conservative government and reporting under a Liberal government, it was perceived as a bipartisan committee.[22]

Second, while progressive forces were able to take control of the Liberal Party when it was in opposition, there was a right-wing revival inside the party upon its reelection in 1962. This revival took place under the leadership of Mitchell Sharp, who would become minister of finance in 1965. Sharp was philosophically opposed to expanding public medical care insurance and felt that, if it had to be done, it was best to limit federal involvement to a cost-sharing basis.[23]

Third, even though the Liberal party had firmly committed to moving forward on medical care insurance before the Saskatchewan plan was implemented, this development was critical in prompting a shift away from a straight federal program.[24] Displacing an existing provincial program would be politically much more difficult in terms of federal–provincial relations than simply sharing the costs for eligible provincial programs. Ironically, the successful reform in Saskatchewan made a straight federal program of physician care insurance (whether universal or categorical such as a program limited to children) significantly more difficult politically.

Electoral considerations figured prominently in the final formulation of the federal proposals. By 1965, the government was "frayed" by pension and flag debates and felt that the root of the problem was its status as a minority government.[25] As pressure within the Liberal government to go to an election built, there was also a strong belief that the party needed a well-defined medical care insurance proposal to successfully wage an election campaign. In light of the various factors outlined above, the proposal that emerged was for federal cost-sharing of provincial programs of medical care insurance. The nation-building intent behind the program, however, remained implicit. The Liberal electoral strategy can be summed up in the words of senior Liberal strategist Walter Gordon: "We should appeal for a strong federal government to build a new Canada. We should request a mandate to proceed with such programs as Medicare. . . . it would be a mistake to emphasize the Québec problem, not because we do not consider it the number-one domestic issue but because people in English-speaking Canada do not like being reminded of it" (Gordon 1977, 224).

As Kent outlines, the role of Québec was "absolutely crucial" to the endorsement of medical care insurance by the federal government: "There would have been no Canadian welfare state if pre-1960 Québec politics had continued."[26] Changes in Québec were "absolutely essential to moving ahead." The new Lésage government was as keen on social policy as was the federal Liberal government. Federal officials perceived the Pearson government and Lésage government of Québec as having the same broad objectives in health care, and federal officials believed that a federal cost-sharing program could be made politically acceptable even in light of Québec nationalism. In so doing, the federal cost-sharing proposal for medical care was significantly different from cost-sharing for hospital care, with the former being based on broad principles rather than federal monitoring of a detailed program. Federal policymakers fashioned a proposal that proved impossible for the Liberal government in Québec to resist.

As soon as the federal government announced its intentions to initiate a federal cost-sharing program for medical care insurance, the Québec government declared that it intended to bring in its own program outside the rubric of any federal shared-cost plan (Taylor 1987, 356). To this point, there had been very little government action in Québec to support this claim. It was after the conference that the Québec premier "set events in motion," announcing that health insurance would be introduced the following year and establishing a committee to study the issue (Taylor 1987, 386, 392). The two governments now were jockeying to be the first to occupy the political space created by the issue of medical care insurance—engaging in competitive state-building, to use Banting's apt phrase.

Although the Liberal government in Québec was replaced by the Union Natio-nale government in mid-1966, the Québec government continued to insist that it had full jurisdictional competence over health care and demanded that the federal government cede further tax room and return to Québec the tax capacity that it required to exercise this competence (Taylor 1987, 386). Despite the fact that the influential Castonguay committee (which had been appointed by the Québec Liber-als) recommended the establishment of a comprehensive, universal provincial health insurance program, the Union Nationale publicly committed itself to a policy of subsidizing health insurance provided to those with low income through existing agencies (Taylor 1987, 389–90).

Two factors combined to make this policy position futile. First, the structure of the federal "health insurance tax" meant that even if the Québec government were to refuse to go along with the federal plan, Québec citizens would still be taxed and the proceeds transferred to other provinces. Of course the Québec government (and some Québec members of parliament) vociferously protested against the federal position; however, the federal government, from the outset, refused to budge. As the national program was implemented and Québec stayed out, federal intransi-gence was reinforced by the election results of 1968: "The federal government with its recently acquired large majority in the Commons, and especially its success in Quebec, was in no mood to compromise" (Taylor 1987, 392). Second, the position of the Québec government ran against strong public support for medicare inside the province of Québec—a factor that the federal government was counting on. Support for the federal medicare program in Québec proved to be higher than in any other region in Canada by a considerable margin (see table 8.2).

Given the immense pressure on the Québec provincial government generated by federal maneuvering, it seemed largely a foregone conclusion that Québec would

Table 8.2 Support for Medicare, Canada, by Region, 1968 (Percentage)

	National	Québec	Ontario	West
Federal government should bring in:				
Medicare as promised	55	64	49	55
Medicare should be postponed	19	20	19	19
Medicare should be dropped	19	12	23	19
Can't say	7	4	9	7

Source: Taylor 1987, 391.

eventually join the program despite its efforts to resist (Taylor 1990, 150).[27] Regardless of aspirations to exercise full provincial autonomy, the Québec government could not resist the federal offer even in the face of federally stipulated "national principles."

Implementing Medical Care Insurance in Québec

Responding to federal pressure to adopt a compulsory universal insurance program for medical care thrust the Québec government into a serious confrontation with powerful political forces within its own province—a confrontation that ultimately had momentous repercussions for the development of health care in Canada. On one side was the medical profession. In the Québec case the profession was split, and while the general practitioners supported the principle of universal medical care insurance, the specialists adamantly believed government intervention should be limited to the subsidization of those unable to afford private insurance. On the other side were forces united in a "common front," including labor unions, teachers, and farmers, calling for a system of state medicine like the British NHS with salaried doctors and a crown corporation to manufacture and distribute pharmaceuticals (Taylor 1987, 397).

As it became clear that the provincial government would move ahead with public medical care insurance, the "common front" attacked the Union Nationale's legislation, which would allow a certain number of specialists to opt out of the program with financial compensation (that is, allowing them to extra-bill) as "perpetuating the privilèges intolérables of the doctors" and threatened their own strike if the provision was not removed (Taylor 1987, 397, 400).[28] In the face of this pressure, the government removed the provision for opting out with financial compensation—effectively banning the practice of extra-billing in Québec.

The specialists went on strike (though emergency specialist services were maintained) and were legislated back to work in the dramatic context of the FLQ crisis.[29] As Taylor notes,

> It was the Quebec sub-plot, however, that was to become the most conflict-ridden, and therefore the most politically perilous, of all. Commencing with a disagreement with the federal government, it rose to crisis proportions with the specialists'

withdrawal of services, and reached its climax as medicare became inextricably bound up with, and its dénouement greatly influenced by, an even greater crisis—the kidnapping of a foreign diplomat, murder of a Cabinet minister, and a federal government finding of "apprehended insurrection." It surpassed in magnitude even the crisis of Saskatchewan eight years earlier. (Taylor 1987, 379).

The final outcome was that extra-billing and user fees were, contrary to the situation in the nine English-speaking provinces, banned under the provincial medical insurance plan. As argued in the next section, this situation set the stage for the advent of federal legislation in the form of the CHA.

The Consolidation of Public Health Insurance in Canada, 1971–86

Important changes were to take place in the federal program for cost-sharing hospital and medical care insurance in Canada in the decade and a half following the implementation of a complete set of provincial medical care insurance programs in 1971. The first was the shifting of the matching cost-sharing grants for hospital and medical care to a block-funding formula under the Establish Programs Financing (EPF) arrangements in 1977. At the same time and, in part as a result of this change, federal principles in public health insurance came to be seen as eroding. In conjunction with the serious challenge to the integrity of the Canadian state posed by the political success of the sovereignty movement in Québec in the latter half of the 1970s, these factors resulted in the CHA. The latter was designed to reinforce (and tighten up) the standards governing federal transfers to the provinces for public health insurance. This legislation significantly reinforced the existing system of universal, first-dollar public health insurance in coverage and set the stage for the development of public health insurance's iconic status in Canada.

Financing Canadian Health Insurance—Established Programs Financing

Cost-sharing programs posed a serious difficulty from the federal perspective—the federal government retained no measure of direct control over its own costs for these programs. As a response, in 1976 the federal government proposed ending the matching cost-sharing arrangements for hospital and medical care insurance as well as for postsecondary education. Instead, the federal government proposed to transfer 12.5 percentage points of personal income tax (13.5 was the final settlement) and 1 percentage point of corporate income tax by providing "tax room" (lowering federal taxes) that the provincial governments could then occupy by commensurately increasing their own tax rates. The amount of tax room offered was calculated to approximate one-half of the current federal contribution for the three programs and the remainder would continue to be provided in cash.[30] At least in the short term, these arrangements seemed to satisfy both the federal and provincial governments. The shift to established programs financing (EPF) brought stability to federal expenditures. For their part, provinces were now fully exposed to the risk of cost increases greater than GDP growth, but at the same time, EPF provided them with greater flexibility in determining how to allocate health care expenditures.

No sooner had these changes come into force than the ability of the federal government to maintain the national principles attached to hospital and medical care insurance was brought into question. By the late 1970s the federal government was increasingly facing charges that it was allowing the national principles underpinning hospital and medical care insurance to erode. Of central concern was the issue of extra-billing by which various provinces such Alberta and Ontario were allowing physicians to charge patients fees over and above those received under the provincial insurance plan. These practices were generating considerable public concern.[31] The federal government set up a commission headed by Justice Emmett Hall (who had headed the royal commission in the early 1960s that initially proposed universal comprehensive health insurance.) The terms of reference for the Hall Commission were twofold: to determine whether federal funds were being diverted to nonhealth purposes and to determine whether extra-billing and user fees were contravening the principle of "reasonable access" (Taylor 1990, 159). On the first question, the finding was that provinces were not diverting federal funds. On the second question, the commission report was adamant that user charges were posing serious impediments to reasonable access.[32] As outlined earlier, in contrast to most other provinces, Québec had banned extra-billing from the inception of its program. As a result of this discrepancy the focus given to impediments to "reasonable access" to health services caused by extra-billing and user fees in various English Canadian provinces was particularly politically awkward for the federal government.

Enforcing a National Program—The Canada Health Act (1984)

Public health insurance in Canada continued to be caught up in the territorial politics of the Canadian federation—dynamics that were particularly powerful in the period surrounding the 1980 referendum in Québec on sovereignty-association. One of the primary federal strategies in the Québec referendum was to argue that continued federal involvement was required to maintain the standards of social programs in Québec. As the leader of NDP at the time, Ed Broadbent, later noted: "In the 1980 referendum, Prime Minister Pierre Trudeau could honestly point to Ottawa as the source and guarantor of popular programs like unemployment insurance, health care and pensions."[33] During the referendum debate, federal ministers argued that "a sovereign Quebec would not be able to sustain the social programs that Quebecers enjoyed as citizens of Canada" (Banting 1995, 287).[34] The federal government could hardly claim responsibility, however, for maintaining the standard of public health insurance provision in Québec when these standards were demonstrably more stringent than those enforced by the federal government, as evident by the state of public health insurance in a number of the English-speaking provinces.

The accommodating approach that had guided federal health care funding reforms in the mid-1970s was replaced by a new, more forceful approach when the

Liberals, having been replaced by a Conservative minority government in 1979, again formed the government in February 1980. Coincidentally the Québec referendum was set for May 1980. During the federal election campaign of 1980, which also had important implications for the playing out of the "Non" campaign in the Québec referendum, the former federal Minister of Health Monique Bégin vigorously attacked extra-billing and user fees and promised to end both practices if elected (Taylor 1990, 167). Immediately upon her reappointment as minister of health following the Liberal success in the 1980 election, senior departmental officials immediately began preparing a strategy to deal with this problem.

Thus the CHA had its genesis in federal involvement in the Québec referendum campaign. The federal government's decision to move to EPF in 1976, which has been described as "the most massive transfer of revenues (and therefore substance of power) from the federal to the provincial governments in Canadian history," not only failed to stem separatist sentiment in Québec but also, by 1980, represented a significant political liability (Taylor 1990, 166). In the wake of the failed referendum, the federal government seized the opportunity to reverse the developments precipitated by the move to EPF and shore up its position vis-à-vis the provinces with the CHA.

Repositioning itself in the area of public health insurance was strongly in keeping with a number of other initiatives designed to rebalance the locus of power in the federation in the wake of the Québec referendum. The most visible of these efforts was the patriation of the Canadian constitution following lengthy and complex negotiations with the provinces.[35] Central in the constitutional exercise was the creation of the Canadian Charter of Rights and Freedoms, which replaced the Canadian Bill of Rights (which was only federal legislation). The intent was to strengthen the rights inherent in national citizenship—to which the intent of the CHA to strengthen the social rights inherent in national citizenship was analogous.[36]

In 1984 the federal government adopted the Canada Health Act. The CHA replaced legislation for the existing programs of hospital insurance and medical care insurance as well as restated, clarified, and tightened up the conditions of the two existing programs. Five federally defined national principles made up the core of the CHA:

- Public administration (each provincial plan must be run by a nonprofit, public authority accountable to the provincial government);
- Comprehensiveness (provinces must provide coverage for all necessary physician and hospital services);
- Universality (insured services must be universally available to all residents of the province under uniform terms and conditions with waiting periods for new entrants being limited to a maximum of three months);
- Portability (each provincial plan must be portable so that eligible residents are covered while they are temporarily out of the province); and
- Accessibility (reasonable access to insured services is not to be impaired by charges or other mechanisms, and reasonable compensation must be made to physicians for providing insured services).

Application of penalties for violation of these five federally defined principles remained discretionary.

Crucially, however, the CHA mandated automatic dollar-for-dollar reductions in federal funds for revenue collected in a province through user fees and extra-billing standing in stark contrast to the discretionary application of the five principles.[37] This discrepancy had three major effects. First, it brought the practice in the English Canadian provinces in line with existing practice in Québec, which had already banned extra-billing and user fees. Second, although the ban was a central cause of friction with other provinces, it did not generate any friction with Québec as that province was already in compliance with the nondiscretionary elements of the legislation. Third, by allowing for discretionary application of all other requirements, the legislation maximized the federal government's latitude to relax future application of the CHA in Québec rather than potentially forcing the federal government into future confrontations with that province—a point that, at the time, was likely not lost on Québec officials. For example, Québec later adopted long-standing practices in violation of the CHA that the federal government would simply never enforce.[38]

To the medical profession and provincial governments, the CHA represented "an unwarranted, powerful and, for the provincial governments, politically hazardous federal intrusion into a field of provincial jurisdiction" (Taylor 1990, 166). The provinces faced the difficult choice of whether to allow their physicians to extra-bill and incur the penalty in terms of reduced federal transfers or be forced into a confrontation with the medical profession, which was staunchly opposed to the ban. In some cases, such as Alberta, the government fervently defended the right of providers to extra-bill and banned the practice only under duress. In other cases serious confrontations developed between provincial governments and the medical profession. Conflict was most serious in the case of Ontario where provincial compliance with the federal legislation precipitated the third provincial doctors' strike in Canada in a twenty-five-year period. Although it was clear well before the strike that the government would be able to garner almost unanimous legislative support to legislate doctors back to work, the OMA itself aborted the strike after twenty-five days, acknowledging its own "failure to reach the public" (Taylor 1990, 175).

Despite some provincial protestation, especially from Alberta, British Columbia, and Ontario, no province could politically afford to allow extra-billing—revealing just how powerful federal conditionality could be in operation. As Guest notes: "Only three provinces, Newfoundland, Prince Edward Island, and Nova Scotia, had eliminated extra-billing and hospital user charges by 30 June 1984. The remaining seven began incurring penalties estimated at $9.5 million a month in July 1984, but before the three years had elapsed, all provinces and territories had ended extra-billing" (1997, 212). The federal government had triumphed in bringing all provinces into line with the practice in Québec and, as a result, reestablished its ability to claim the mantle of the guarantor of national social citizenship rights without having to provoke a direct confrontation with Québec.

Conclusion

A number of comparative examinations of public health insurance in the United States and Canada point to developments in the Canadian provinces as being central in the development of national health insurance north of the border—emphasizing, by way of contrast, the operation of American federalism and the failure of state-level reform to succeed and, in turn, spur federal reform. In contrast with this image of significant differences in the effects of federalism in the United States and Canada, it was argued earlier that federal arrangements had a similarly dampening effect on state and provincial reforms in both countries in earlier periods. Developments in Canada in the medicare era emphasize, moreover, the limited degree to which provincial reforms—even where they emerged—contributed to a national level program. In the Canadian case the implementation of a national program for universal medical care coverage required a much more powerful engine—an engine that was provided by the politics of territorial integration.

In contrast to interpretations that see the emergence of universal, first-dollar coverage as reflecting a distinctive Canadian political culture or set of political institutions relative to those of the United States (with its own distinctive political culture and institutions explaining American exceptionalism), central elements of the Canadian system as it actually emerged—such as the effective banning of extra-billing and user fees in the mid-1980s—were the result of the politics of territorial integration. These elements, which had not been conceived as central to the Canadian system of public health insurance, were grafted onto the system as a result of the complex political interplay centered on territorial integration. Despite their incidental origins, these elements later came to be widely acknowledged as defining characteristics of public health insurance in Canada—highlighting the degree to which public programs can generate their own patterns of supportive public opinion and, more generally, the degree to which policy can shape politics.

CHAPTER NINE

The Iconic Status of Health Care in Canada, 1984–2008

There is simply no other issue of such vital significance to Canadians. . . .
Nowhere does government interact with people in a more meaningful and consequential way.

Liberal Party of Canada, Election Campaign Platform 2004

THE STRATEGY TO USE the national health insurance framework as a
touchstone for citizen identification with the federal government proved
stunningly successful—even if this success was more evident, as we shall see, outside
of Québec than within. Public health insurance was transformed into an icon of
national citizenship as well as an emblem of Canadian distinctiveness vis-à-vis the
United States—most powerfully in the English-speaking provinces. In the 1990s the
federal role languished as the federal government targeted health care transfers to
achieve its goals of budgetary restraint. Following the near victory of secessionist
forces in the Québec referendum of 1995, however, the federal government began
a vigorous campaign to reassert federal leadership in health care—first through
proposals to expand national programs for universal public coverage to areas such
as prescription drug and home care and later through proposals to consolidate the
existing system of public health insurance for hospital and medical care insurance
through wait-time guarantees. Through this, territorial politics remained central in
the politics of public health insurance.

National Unity and National Distinctiveness

Support for public health insurance became increasingly strongly linked to issues of
national unity as well as Canadian distinctiveness. In a 1978 poll, 72 percent of
respondents agreed that medical care "should be guaranteed by the government"
(Mendelsohn 2001, 28). By 1985, 95 percent of Canadian respondents agreed. In
1965, 52 percent of people responding to a poll favored a voluntary plan while only
41 percent favored a universal plan, and in 1968, only 55 percent of respondents

(and less than half in Ontario) felt that the federal government should bring in Medicare as it had promised (Taylor 1987, 391). In contrast, by 2000, 88 percent of respondents said that it was "very important" to them to have a "strong national system of publicly funded health care"—only 3 percent felt it was "not important" (Mendelsohn 2001, 25). As Marmor and coauthors noted: "None of the major studies of the origins of Medicare [in Canada] . . . have concluded that the overwhelming support for the egalitarian values of the Medicare program preceded the passage of national health insurance legislation." Rather, "the values expressed by the . . . operating principles of Medicare . . . have in large measure arisen from Medicare's performance, not its origins" (Marmor, Okma, and Latham 2002, 16). Public support for the program is not explained solely by its performance, however. These shifts were also related to public perceptions of the role of health insurance in fostering national unity and defining a national identity precisely as intended, though to a degree not anticipated by, federal policymakers.

Public Health Insurance, Citizenship, and National Unity

Public health insurance has come to be seen in Canada as a right of citizenship. In a 1998 poll 69 percent of respondents agreed (48 percent agreed "completely") and only 11 percent of respondents disagreed that "Medicare is a right of citizenship" (Mendelsohn 2001, 28). Perceived in this way, health care fosters national unity by defining the national community as the community through which this right is granted. The central principles of the CHA, especially universal coverage, equal access, and cross-provincial portability of benefits, "have come to define the citizenship dimensions of health provision in Canada" (Maioni 2002). When asked in a 1994 poll to identify what "most ties us together as a nation," the two responses garnering substantial agreement were health care and hockey (Stanbury 1996).

The corollary of perceiving health care as a right is the demand for a high degree of national uniformity in the provision of public health services. The degree of provincial variability that is politically acceptable in delivering a service that is a right of national citizenship is necessarily limited. In a 1996 poll 63 percent of respondents felt that it was "very essential" to have national standards for health care across the country while another 25 percent felt it was somewhat essential (Mendelsohn 2001, 80).[1]

The federal role in health care through its link with citizenship is imbued with considerable symbolic significance. As Maioni puts it:

> The federal government can claim to have "nationalized" health care and promoted "equal citizenship" among Canadians and guaranteed health benefits to all. In debates about provincial autonomy, national unity, or constitutional renewal, this is of enormous significance: the federal government has no constitutional role in health care but can claim to defend the "integrity" of the popular features of the "Canadian" health care model. The federal government achieves clout without the headache of administering and budgeting for health care services. (2001, 100)

All relevant political actors "recognize the extent to which disputes about health care involve struggles over economic and political space in the federation" (2001, 88).

Public Health Insurance and Canadian Distinctiveness

Public health insurance has also become a central defining element of Canadian distinctiveness as a result of its role in debates regarding free trade between the United States and Canada. No sooner had the CHA passed than the Conservative government under Prime Minister Brian Mulroney officially announced free trade talks with the United States—a proposal that received quick and enthusiastic support from President Ronald Reagan. Congress then gave the president time-limited authority to conclude a free trade agreement with Canada. Negotiations took place over the next two years with the agreement being signed in early 1988. In a rare display of its power, the unelected Canadian Senate refused to ratify the agreement unless the Conservative government received public support for the deal in a general election. Free trade with the United States dominated the Canadian election of 1988, which the governing Conservatives won by a strong margin with 43 percent of the popular vote in comparison with the Liberal Opposition's 31.9 percent.

The issue of free trade had prompted a widespread public debate about the potential risks to Canada's national identity posed by deepening trade relations with the United States. Although publicly provided services were not formally included in the negotiations, public health insurance became central to this debate. Barbara McDougall, who served as secretary of state for external affairs in the Progressive Conservative government from 1991 to 1993, summarized the anxiety in a 2001 speech:

> Critics argued that harmonization pressures would inevitably result from entering into an agreement with the US, creating *de facto* pressures, if not *de jure* ones. In order to remain competitive with US firms, it was argued that Canadian firms would have to liberalize social programs which would have the effect of fraying Canada's social safety net, including its valued universal health care system. The negative implications became received wisdom in the public debate. And the feared harmonization effects became a rallying point for those fearing that the unique Canadian social fabric would be shredded and altered to fit the American model.

This debate recurred in 1993 in the face of negotiations regarding the deepening and broadening of continental economic integration under the North American Free Trade Agreement (NAFTA). Capturing an important strain of public debate regarding NAFTA in Canada, Public Citizen argued that NAFTA's "core provisions . . . promote . . . the privatization and deregulation of essential services, such as . . . health care."[2] Publicly provided health services were not broadly excluded from the NAFTA provisions but were protected under specific reservations set out in the annexes to the agreement. In 1996 the three signatory countries signed a letter agreeing that existing provincial health services were "fully protected" under NAFTA (see Canada, Department of Foreign Affairs and International Trade, 1996).

This would not, however, stem concern over the future application of investor protection provisions under Chapter 11 of NAFTA to public health services in Canada (Romanow 2002, 237).[3] A decade later, the Commission on the Future of Health Care in Canada argued that it was necessary "to ensure that the increasing economic interdependence of countries like ours does not compromise our ability to make our own decisions about political, economic and social policies, including health care" (Romanow 2002, 235).

The focus on public health insurance in the debates over free trade significantly reinforced the status of public health insurance as a central element of Canadian national identity. In a 1996 poll a staggering 96 percent of respondents felt that the health care system was important (82 percent responding "very important" and 14 percent responding "somewhat important") to the Canadian identity. In a 1998 poll 72 percent of respondents agreed (52 percent completely agree, 20 percent agree) that "Medicare embodies Canadian values" while only 9 percent disagreed (Mendelsohn 2001, 27–28).

Ironically globalization, continental economic integration, and the resulting constraints on public policy have, concomitantly, strengthened public health care in Canada. Canadian governments are increasingly restricted (or have increasingly chosen to restrict themselves) in a number of key areas: monetary policy (with the adoption of a permanent policy of low inflation), fiscal policy (with a movement away from Keynesianism in favor of balanced budgets and permanent austerity), trade policy (with tariff options increasingly being restricted by international trade agreements), industrial policy and regional development policy (with subsidies also being increasingly restricted by international trade agreements), and taxation policy (with an ongoing commitment to competitive corporate tax rates especially relative to the United States). These constraints have operated most powerfully vis-à-vis the federal government. They have been less restrictive in regard to functions typically exercised by provincial governments: provision of education, postsecondary education, health care, and municipal services.

At the same time health care is one of the main areas of federal activity that remains relatively unconstrained by international agreements or concerns about international competitiveness. As a result health care has become more and more central to how the federal government in Canada defines its function. This has contributed to health care becoming the dominant focus of federal–provincial relations and a central issue in each of the past four federal general elections over the last decade.

The Elevation of Health Care to Quasi-Constitutional Status

From the mid-1990s to the present, health care has become the central focus of intergovernmental interaction in Canada—displacing the pride of place formerly enjoyed by constitutional issues. The recent spate of health accords from 1999 to 2004 in Canada have been matters of top-level interprovincial negotiations and signed by first ministers themselves. Arguably, twenty years ago, intergovernmental agreements at comparable levels of detail would have been a matter for ministers responsible for health. The elevation of health care to quasi-constitutional status has been the result of a number of trends: the increasing centrality of health care to the role of the federal government as discussed above, the increasing political popularity of health care and popular concern with health care as an issue, and finally, a deliberate strategy by the federal government to focus federal–provincial relations on functional rather than on constitutional issues.

The centrality of constitutional issues in intergovernmental relations in the decade following the patriation of the Canadian constitution in 1982 resulted from the fact that Québec did not sign the Canadian Constitution Act as agreed to by the federal government and nine other provinces in 1982 although the province would be bound by it. This created an ongoing constitutional dilemma in Canada that engendered several attempts to resolve this situation. The first attempt to bring Québec back into the constitutional fold, the Meech Lake Accord, was agreed to in 1987 by the federal government and all ten provinces. However, the accord failed to receive subsequent legislative ratification in two provinces and expired in 1990. A second attempt culminated in the Charlottetown Agreement in 1992. This package of reforms was put to a national referendum, which it failed to pass. The failure of both constitutional agreements had been significant political losses for the federal Progressive Conservative government under Prime Minister Brian Mulroney.

Upon coming to power in 1993, the new Liberal government under Prime Minister Jean Chrétien was committed to not reopening constitutional discussions. Rather the government's strategy was to weaken support for sovereignty in Québec, not through constitutional negotiations, but by demonstrating how well Canadian federalism could work by focusing on functional areas of federal–provincial interaction including health care. This strategy, to which the federal government has since hewn under the leadership of various prime ministers and parties, has had the concomitant effect of creating a vacuum in federal–provincial relations at the senior—including first ministers—level.

In combination with the other factors outlined, the result has been that intergovernmental relations at the most senior levels in Canada are no longer dominated by constitutional issues (or broader issues regarding the overall direction of the Canadian federation) and that, at least from the late 1990s until the mid-2000s, health care has come to fill the void. The result has been that the politics of health care are now aptly described as an increasingly sophisticated "political football game" that is "played by professional state-builders in a charged atmosphere in which the political and financial stakes are considerably higher than they were in the past" (Maioni 2001, 87).

Federal Efforts at Reform

A decade after the inception of the CHA, the federal government began more than a decade of efforts to reinvigorate its role in health care. These federal attempts at health care reform from 1995 to the present illustrate the embeddedness of public health insurance in the public consciousness, the rise of health care to quasi-constitutional status, and the need for the federal government to again draw on health care as means of territorial integration in the face of concerns regarding the territorial integrity of the Canadian federation precipitated by the Québec referendum on secession in October 1995.

Federal Transfer Restructuring

The February 1995 federal budget stunned the provinces with the announcement of the most significant change in federal health care policy in over a decade. Without prior consultation with the provinces, the federal government announced that its contribution to funding for public hospital and medical care insurance would be rolled into a single block transfer for all health and social services under the Canada Health and Social Transfer (CHST)—marking a large, sudden, and unanticipated policy shift. Most important, the shift to the CHST would be accompanied by a significant reduction in federal transfers (see figure 9.1). Pressures on fiscal arrangements had begun to build when, with the CHA not even fully implemented in the provinces, the federal government began to restrict growth in transfers. Growth in EPF transfers were increasingly restricted (indexed to gross national product growth minus 2 percent in 1986 and further restricted to GNP growth minus 3 percent in 1989) and frozen in the early 1990s. It was the shift from EPF to the CHST, however, that signaled the full extent to which the federal government would attempt to retract its financial commitment to public health insurance.

Figure 9.1   Federal Cash Transfers to Provinces for Health Care, Canada, 1993–2007

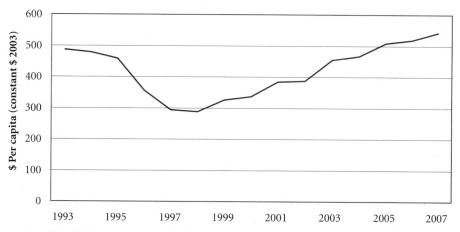

Sources and Notes: Federal cash transfers for health from 1993 to 2003–04 are calculated as 62% of actual CHST cash transfers (using the Department of Finance estimate of the proportion of GST going to health.) Federal cash transfers for health after 2004 are comprised of the cash component of the Canada Health Transfer. (CHT)

Transfers per capita were calculated by the author using population data from CANSIM I Matrix 00001. Adjustment of transfers per capita to constant dollars (2003) was calculated by the author using CANSIM 1 Series P100000 and CANSIM II Series V735319. Constant dollars for 2004–2007 are estimated using the three-year average CPI increase for 2000–2003. Population figures for 2004–2007 are estimated from Statistics Canada population projections, CANSIM II, Table 052–0001.

The federal government appeared to believe that CHA's robust political popularity would allow it to reduce its financial contribution to provincial health care programs without threatening the integrity of those programs. While the Canada Health Act would still be in effect, however, it was unclear how the federal government would enforce its provisions, considering that the cash portion of the new CHST was scheduled to be displaced by tax point transfers over the next decade.[4] At the same time, the federal government engaged in a number of skirmishes with the provinces over violations of the CHA provisions regarding user fees and extra-billing in an apparent attempt to demonstrate that it would still have sufficient financial muscle under the new arrangements to enforce the CHA.[5] Federal policy-makers did not seem to perceive at the time just how close they were to a near-death experience.

The Québec Referendum

On October 31, 1995, 93 percent of Québec voters cast votes in a provincial referendum on whether Québec should "become sovereign." The outcome, in which the votes of just over one-half of 1 percent of voters allowed the "non" side the smallest imaginable margin of victory, represented the most serious challenge to the territorial integrity of the Canadian state since Confederation. Numerous charges were launched inside and outside Québec that the federal government had been sleepwalking through the referendum campaign and that federal leadership was clearly to blame for the near victory of secessionist forces.

Having narrowly averted defeat, the federal government put in motion a two-pronged strategy of response: Plan A to demonstrate to Québec that its demands could be accommodated within the confines of the existing Canadian federal system and the infamous Plan B, a strategy to more directly challenge those advocating Québec sovereignty. The latter entailed a reference case submitted to the Supreme Court of Canada to consider the conditions under which Québec could legally begin negotiations to secede from the Canadian federation, which federalists had claimed the sovereignists had soft-pedaled during the referendum campaign. In terms of the former, the visibility of the federal role in all social programs—but especially public health insurance—became even more critical.

Reinvigorating the Federal Role, 1997–2008

Federal efforts at reform in the decade following the Québec referendum highlight the degree to which health care in Canada has captured the focus of political officials at the highest level, achieved a quasi-constitutional status, and come to dominate electoral politics in Canada while, at the same time, continuing to be inextricably intertwined with the politics of territorial integration.

In the 1997 election, the first following the Québec referendum, the Liberals proposed a number of ambitious reforms to reinvigorate the federal role in public health care. Health care had only been a minor issue in the federal election of 1993 (in which the Liberal government replaced the Conservative government of Brian Mulroney, which had held power for nine years) although the Liberals had committed to forming a major commission (the National Forum on Health) to study the health care system (Liberal Party 1993, 81).[6] The Liberal Party platform in the next election in 1997 echoed the forum's recommendations regarding changes in funding for primary care, home care, and prescription drugs and, most notably, committed to the development of a "a timetable and fiscal framework for the implementation of universal public coverage for medically necessary prescription drugs" (Liberal Party 1997, 72, 75).

For the most part, these reforms were not achieved. Rather, in response to intense provincial pressure to restore federal funding, federal initiatives in the late 1990s were largely limited to reinjecting cash and reinforcing the federal–provincial commitment to the principles of the CHA. As a good example of this, the Social Union Framework Agreement (SUFA) of February 1999, struck between the federal government and the provincial/territorial governments (with the exception of Quebec), provided enriched funding for health care but little substantive change. In this agreement, the federal government increased the cash component of the CHST and agreed to limitations on the federal spending power in terms of establishing new cost-shared programs (Canada, Department of Finance 1999). Provincial governments, in turn, committed themselves to respecting the principles of the CHA and provided assurances that they would spend the increased transfers on health care.

Nevertheless, the federal government continued its attempts to expand public health insurance coverage. Less than a year later, the federal minister of health announced a new plan to "save" Canada's health care system in January 2000 that included, among other things, a major new matching cost-sharing initiative for home care. Less than six months later, the home care plan was officially dead in the face of provincial resistance.

Health care also was a central issue in the November 2000 federal general election. The Liberal election platform in 2000 committed the Liberal government to protecting against the development of "two-tier" health care (typically taken in Canada to mean user fees and extra-billing) (Liberal Party 2000, 15). Upon being returned to office, the Liberal government announced the formation of the Royal Commission on the Future of Health Care in Canada—the Romanow Commission. The commission was to report at the same time as the Senate Committee on Social Affairs, Science, and Technology under the chair of Senator Michael Kirby (the Kirby Committee), which had been studying the health care system since late 1999. Both reports suggested a strong reinvigoration of the federal role in health, strengthening federal transfers to the provinces, reinforcing national principles of medicare as enshrined in the CHA, and new programs for federal–provincial matching conditional cost-sharing, including programs for catastrophic drug coverage, home care, and primary care reform.

In response, the federal government entered a new round of negotiations with the provinces, and in February 2003, the prime minister and premiers announced the Health Care Renewal Accord of 2003. The accord restated the five principles of the CHA with a renewed focus (also emphasized in the Health Accord 2000) on timeliness of access, quality of services, and sustainability of the system.[7] The main thrust of the accord in terms of public health insurance coverage was the extension of public health insurance to home care and catastrophic drug care with the prime minister and premiers committing themselves to "ensure that Canadians, wherever they live, have reasonable access to catastrophic drug coverage" by the end of 2005–6 (Health Canada 2003).

Despite the fact that the Health Care Renewal Accord was signed less than a year earlier, the new Liberal prime minister, Paul Martin announced in March 2004 that he would seek an agreement with the provinces for a ten-year plan for the Canadian health care system and, calling an election for June 2004, claimed that he needed an electoral mandate in order to strike a deal with the provinces on health care (Clark 2004). The ensuing campaign again demonstrated the centrality of health care to federal electoral politics as well as the degree to which partisan consensus on health care had emerged in response to popular support for the existing system enshrined in the CHA. From the outset, the primary electoral strategy of the Liberals was to focus on the issue of health care in order to exploit differences between the Liberals and the resurgent Conservative Party of Canada (CPC) and the perceived weakness of the latter on the issue of health care.[8]

The Liberal campaign platform included reform to primary health care, a reduction in waiting times, a comprehensive strategy to increase support for informal caregivers and a National Home Care Program that would allocate money on a per capita basis to provinces meeting a minimum, agreed-upon set of home care services. In the area of prescription drugs, the Liberal Party committed to a "nationwide approach to provide all Canadians with a basic level of coverage, including catastrophic protection" by first agreeing to a "national pharmaceuticals strategy" by 2006, which would be followed by enacting legislation and establishing a federal funding contribution (Liberal Party 2004, 22). The three major national parties (the Liberals, Conservatives, and New Democratic Party) demonstrated a significant degree of consensus on the issue of health care with each committing to defend the principles of the CHA, to devote greater resources to the area of health care, and to expand public health insurance coverage. Ultimately, the minor differences between the major national parties over health care played little role in the election outcome, and the Liberals were returned as a relatively weak minority government.

Prime Minister Martin's focus on health care reform as the reason for calling an election necessitated subsequent federal–provincial negotiations in which the extension of public health insurance coverage again arose as a possibility. The agreement also restated the commitment made in the 2003 Health Accord to provide first-dollar coverage by 2006 for short-term acute home care (two weeks), short-term acute community mental health (two weeks), and end-of-life care.[9] The deal also injected considerable new federal money into transfers for health care and placed transfers on a stable basis by including a fixed escalator of 6 percent. In figure 9.2 are the projected figures for CHT through 2014, including new transfers. Significant expansion of public insurance coverage would not be part of the final deal, however, as the federal and provincial governments could not agree on terms for expanded public pharmaceutical coverage. In the end the first ministers committed themselves only to "develop, assess, and cost options for catastrophic pharmaceutical coverage."[10] Nevertheless, the federal government continued to struggle to reinvigorate its role in the provision of health services in Canada.

Figure 9.2   Canada Health Transfers, 2004–14

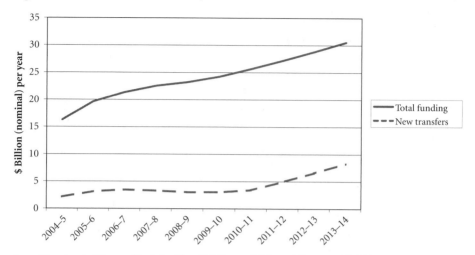

Source: Department of Finance, *The Budget Plan, 2005* (Ottawa: Minister of Finance, 2005), Table 3.1, 70.

The Health Care Issue in Québec

A concern with the role of federal social programs as tools of territorial integration similar to that which motivated federal reformers more than forty years before remained evident in these debates. Former Liberal Party pollster Martin Goldfarb (2004) captured the essence of these concerns:

> The federal government has few direct touch points with individual Canadians. So whenever it has an opportunity to deal directly with its citizens, it should do so, to increase the federal government's relevance to their daily lives. The more Ottawa becomes involved with Canadians, the more individuals are likely to see the value of the national government, nationalism and our federation. One way to accomplish these goals is with a national pharmacare program.

Another aspect related to the territorial dimensions of the health care issue has been the reticence of the federal government to impose federal principles on the delivery of health care in Québec. One of the more revealing aspects of the 2004 negotiations to "fix health care for a generation" was that the private delivery of publicly funded health care, the issue that had most animated Prime Minister Martin during the election campaign, was simply not on the table—not even open for discussion (Curry 2004). The reason for this absence was the need to secure the agreement of the Québec government in a context in which any direct federal attack on privately provided health services could be interpreted as a challenge to Québec's jurisdictional integrity. It was politically rewarding for the federal government to be seen to be standing up to provinces like Alberta in enforcing the principles of the politically popular CHA. To attempt to enforce a federal vision of health care in

Québec in an area of exclusive provincial jurisdiction where federal principles are seen as desirable but not central to notions of identity, creates a serious risk for the federal government and its ability to use health care as a tool of territorial integration.

Perhaps the most important aspect of the 2004 deal was its territorial dimensions. Moving beyond the emergent tradition of "asterisk federalism,"[11] the federal government signed a separate deal with Québec, the thrust of which was outlined in a joint federal–Québec communiqué (Canada, Office of the Prime Minister 2004b). The communiqué essentially restated in sharper language the emphasis on jurisdictional flexibility in the broader agreement. While there was nothing in the Québec side agreement that was not substantively available to all provinces under the general agreement, the symbolic language was striking and included a formal recognition of the principle of asymmetrical federalism—in the words of the communiqué, "flexible federalism that notably allows for the existence of specific agreements and arrangements adapted to Québec's specificity."

The side deal with Québec, arguably, simply recognized the de facto asymmetry in the health care field. Private provision of health services has proceeded the furthest in Québec, which, by that time, boasted the highest number of private diagnostic facilities (MRI, CT, and ultrasound) in the country (Sokoloff 2004).[12] Drawing a comparison with the Quiet Revolution of the early 1960s, a newspaper editorial wondered whether the development of private-delivery health services in Québec represented a "second Quiet Revolution." Another article referred to Québec as a "province of private clinics." Québec's commitment to forging its own path in health service provision was reflected in national headlines: "Don't Push Quebec, PM Warned: Forced Deal Would Backfire."

This asymmetry in the provision of public health services reflects the long-standing reality of asymmetry in the application of the CHA in Québec, which, as argued above, was genetically encoded into the CHA's DNA. The president of the Québec Medical Association noted publicly that the Martin government had vigorously challenged proposed reforms in the rest of Canada (especially reforms proposed by Alberta during the 2004 election) to which it had turned a blind eye in Québec (Sokoloff 2004). In reference to the high-profile confrontations between the premier of Alberta, Ralph Klein, and Prime Minister Martin over proposed reforms in Alberta that might violate the CHA, he pointedly noted: "Mr. Klein has not suggested anything Quebec governments have not been doing for years . . . When you hear Mr. Charest [premier of Québec] and Mr. Klein talk, they are totally on the same wavelength" (Sokoloff 2004).

The asymmetry in the application of the CHA, in turn, reflects an asymmetry in public preferences regarding the private delivery of health services between Québec and the rest of Canada. For example, public opinion is considerably more supportive of private delivery of health care services in Québec (51 percent) than Canadian public opinion in general (42 percent) and much higher than support in certain regions such as Ontario (34 percent) and Atlantic Canada (34 percent) (Mendelsohn 2001, 48). Similarly public opinion is considerably more supportive of allowing people to pay in order to wait a shorter time for health services in Québec (27 percent strongly approving) than in Canada generally (18 percent) and in various regions such as Atlantic Canada (13 percent), BC (13 percent), Alberta (13 percent), and Ontario (14 percent) (Mendelsohn 2001, 55). As the president of the Québec Medical Association noted, "If other provinces tried to set up what we have, they'd have a revolt on their hands. But in Quebec, it's accepted."

Public sentiment in Québec regarding public health insurance helps illustrate the degree to which popular support for public health insurance in English Canada is a function of its relationship with issues of national identity and distinctiveness vis-à-vis the United States: "Universal health coverage is still important to Quebecers, but it's certainly not a defining characteristic of their national identity. In places like Ontario, people talk about the health care system being public like it's a religion. In Quebec, people think differently" (Sokoloff 2004).

The formal recognition of asymmetry poignantly highlights the fundamental tension the federal government has long faced in using health care as a tool of territorial integration. On the one hand, the establishment and protection of relatively uniform access to public health care services outside of Québec is critical to the federal claim to be the guarantor of social rights in Canada. In turn the requirement of national uniformity in health insurance deriving from its status as a right of national citizenship is the federal government's central philosophic justification in enforcing the CHA outside of Québec. On the other hand, the federal government simultaneously risks serious confrontation with the Québec government if it insists on a strict application of the CHA inside Québec—especially in a context where Québec public opinion is diverging further and further from the norms implied under the CHA.

The degree to which the CHA can effectively be used as a tool of territorial integration depends on the flexibility it allows the federal government in managing this tension. The open question is how much substantive asymmetry in health care provision can be allowed before provincial variation is seen by the broader Canadian public as impinging on national rights of social citizenship. A related question raised at the time of the 2004 accord was whether the recognition of asymmetry would weaken the federal government's ability to enforce the CHA outside of Québec should other provinces attempt to challenge it (Dawson 2004; Coyne 2004).

Conclusion

The use of the national health insurance framework to create a bond between individual Canadian citizens and the federal government has been highly successful. Perhaps ironically though, this strategy has been more successful outside than within Québec. This is in large part due to external factors such as the concern in English Canada regarding Canadian distinctiveness in a context of continental integration—concern that has not been mirrored within Québec. Despite this regional variation, the development of national programs for public health insurance in Canada powerfully illustrates the ability of such programs to mold public opinion and generate widespread patterns of public support. Public health insurance did not emerge from a political culture that was necessarily predisposed toward the public provision of health services; however, national programs of public health insurance certainly have created such a political culture in Canada. The Canadian example suggests that arguments that various proposals for health insurance in the United States simply did not or do not fit with existing public opinion often underestimate the ability of programs and policymakers to alter the boundaries of public consensus—an ability of which a number of American observers of health reform are fully cognizant (Beauchamp 1996; Skocpol 1996).

While thus contributing to the embeddedness of the system, the imperatives of territorial integration, which continue to be a central element in the politics of health reform in Canada, also have created significant constraints on health care reform. Despite the fact that its own resistance to change—even tendency toward sclerosis—has generated tremendous pressure on the existing system, exclusive public funding for first-dollar coverage of hospital and physician services is more firmly embedded politically in Canada in 2008 than it was even a decade ago. Debates over private involvement in the health services sector are now virtually limited to the private provision of publicly funded services.[13] This reflects the broad political popularity of the principles enshrined in the Canada Health Act and the increasingly widespread acceptance of public health insurance as a right of citizenship. This latter development has been the result of the use of health care as a tool of territorial statecraft—ends to which it will undoubtedly be turned in the future.

PART IV

Conclusions

CHAPTER TEN

Contemporary Public Health Insurance in the United States and Canada

Many American commentaries on the Canadian experience are, in fact, discussions of an imaginary Canada that resembles in name only the reality in which Canadians live.

Morris C. Barer and Robert G. Evans, "Interpreting Canada"

Is the U.S. system as bad as some Canadians think—or as marvelous as other Canadians claim? The short answers are no, and no.

Theodore R. Marmor, "Suspect Messages"

THE AMERICAN AND CANADIAN health care systems have each played—and continue to play—an important role in health care reform debates across the border. The use of cross-border examples has tended to be highly politicized, and the example of health care in the other country is often held up as an example to be followed or, more usually, as a dire warning. As a result, cross-national commentary in the health care field has often become a matter of "domestic policy-warfare" (Marmor, Okma, and Latham 2002). This has resulted in widespread misperceptions on both sides of the border regarding the two systems. The differences in health care between the United States and Canada are, at once, both subtle and profound. Certainly they are much more complex than typically portrayed in popular discussions, much media coverage, and even some academic analyses.

A consideration of the contemporary health care systems in the two countries as well as their performance highlights themes relating to the development of each as outlined in the preceding chapters. Rather than representing some optimal, abstract solution to the issues posed by health care, the systems were the result of a complex pattern of historical development. In some important instances, the path of development in each country shared important similarities of sequence with the other; yet, each was also shaped by unique forces. Not surprisingly, the emergent systems share important similarities while exhibiting striking differences. The patterns of similarity and difference between them are more complex than had these systems been a more straightforward projection of differences in political culture or distinctive institutional configuration. Moreover, this complex pattern of similarity and difference is mirrored in differences in each system's performance.

The chapter begins by outlining the similarities and differences in the broad frameworks that compose the national systems of health care provision in Canada and the United States—the culmination of the divergent trajectories of development in the two countries. We then compare the actual provision and coverage of health services in the United States and Canada, a comparison that requires being sensitive to the significant variation among Canadian provinces and among American states. Finally, the chapter undertakes a basic assessment of the two systems' performances, arguing that neither system is clearly superior to the other across the major assessment criteria (quality, access, and cost control) and that the varying performance reflects differences in how each country has structured its health care system.

National Health Care Frameworks in Canada and the United States

As outlined in the chapters above, important differences have emerged between the U.S. and Canadian health care frameworks. The Canadian system is based on universal, comprehensive, first-dollar-coverage public insurance for hospital and physician services, the effective proscription of third-party private provision of insurance for these covered services, and a mixture of public and private provision for the remainder of health services comprising roughly half of all health care expenditures. The U.S. system is more fragmented, providing for universal hospital and physician care insurance coverage for those over sixty-five under Medicare (with premiums, copayments, and deductibles) and public health insurance coverage on a needs-tested basis under Medicaid. Under these two programs, public coverage is extended to roughly a quarter of the U.S. population, with the majority of Americans receiving health insurance coverage through employment-based coverage, which is tax subsidized and regulated by the federal and state governments. Coverage varies on a state-to-state basis, from states with quasi-universal coverage to states where very significant portions of the population are left without any health care coverage. The most notable exception in this regard is the state of Massachusetts, where a 2006 law has required all residents to maintain health insurance as of July 1, 2007. The plan provides for subsidized insurance for people earning less than 300 percent of the federal poverty level and low-cost insurance for other residents not eligible for employer-provided insurance.[1]

Despite these differences, as a result of common elements in the sequence of their development, there are also important similarities between the two systems. First, the structure of health service provision is similar: primarily private physician practice on a fee-for-service basis, and a system of voluntary not-for-profit hospitals, although this picture is made more complex by the growth of HMOs in the United States. Second, the role of public health insurance in the United States is significant, and levels of public expenditure on health care in the two countries are similar—being slightly higher on a per capita basis in the United States. Third, in areas that do not fall under universal public insurance coverage in Canada, such as prescription drugs and dental care, the mix of public and private insurance coverage in the two countries is similar.

The Structure of the Canadian System

As outlined above, the Canadian health care system is highly decentralized with the Canadian provinces being granted the preponderance of jurisdictional authority for health care while the federal government has involved itself in the provision of health care through the federal spending power, which underpins the CHA. While the CHA mandates automatic dollar-for-dollar reductions in federal funds for funds collected in a province through user-fees and extra-billing, penalties for violation of the five federally defined principles is discretionary, and to date, no province has been penalized for violating any of the principles outlined in the CHA even though some provinces have been and continue to be in clear violation of various principles (Flood 2002).

Public intervention in health care provision in Canada is not limited to the public *provision* of hospital and physician care insurance but also the effective *proscription* of private third-party provision of insurance for services is covered under the public plan. This is not a requirement of the CHA, but all provinces have adopted some provisions to discourage third-party insurance for publicly insured services. In all provinces except Ontario, physicians are allowed to charge fees directly to patients (at whatever rate the physician determines) provided that they operate completely outside the public insurance system and do not accept any public payment for these services. As a general rule, however, these services cannot be covered by third-party insurance. Six provinces explicitly banned third-party insurance for insured services, although in the case of Québec the Supreme Court of Canada ruled that such bans, in a context of "unreasonably" long wait times, were contrary to the Québec Charter of Human Rights and Freedoms. The court did not rule that the bans were a violation of the Canadian Charter of Rights (Boychuk 2007a). The remaining four have had other, less stringent, restrictions against third-party insurance while not banning it outright. The prohibitions against third-party insurance may, in fact, be the most significant element of public intervention into health care provision in Canada as well as the key difference between health coverage in Canada and the United States.

While widely portrayed as having a universal public health care system, Canada has, in actuality, a public system of universal hospital and physician care insurance. First, the Canadian system is predicated upon public health insurance, which is distinct from public provision of health services. As Evans put it: "Our physicians are predominantly in self-employed fee practice and our hospitals are not-for-profit organizations under more or less independent Boards of Trustees. This system is virtually identical to that in the United States" (2000, 24).

Second, as public universal first-dollar coverage is limited to hospital and physician care, Canada does not have a universal system of health care; rather, it has a universal insurance coverage for hospital and physician care that together cover (at least in terms of expenditures) less than half of the Canadian health care system.[2] Thus, public health insurance coverage in Canada is aptly thought of as "narrow but deep." It covers a relatively narrow range of health services (hospital and physician care), but in these areas virtually all costs are covered by public insurance.

Other sectors of the Canadian health care system are characterized by various types and levels of government involvement. Prescription drugs and dental care, key elements of the overall health care system, are not covered by universal plans, and most insurance coverage is provided by employers, as is the case in the United States: "The mixed funding system in these sectors is much like the "traditional" American approach" (Evans 2000, 25–26). The relative importance of sectors under universal public insurance and those not (e.g., prescription drugs, long-term care, home care) is shifting toward the latter, with expenditures on drugs growing more quickly than other components of health care expenditures. That is, the sectors without universal public insurance are becoming relatively more and more important—a development that has been termed "passive privatization."

The Structure of the U.S. System

As outlined above, primary responsibility for publicly provided health care resides with the U.S. states by virtue of the Tenth Amendment, which states that any powers not constitutionally delegated to the federal government are reserved for the states. A central role for the federal government in health care provision has evolved, however, through its taxing power (e.g., providing tax subsidies for employer-sponsored health insurance coverage), spending power (e.g., making conditional transfers to the states under programs such as Medicaid), and power to regulate interstate commerce (e.g., prohibiting states from regulating health insurance provided by self-insuring employers).

The major form of federal intervention in health care remains health insurance coverage for seniors under Medicare and for low-income individuals under Medicaid. Together the two programs cover approximately a quarter of the population.[3] Under these two programs and other public expenditures for health, public expenditures represent approximately half of total health care expenditures in the United States.

Under Medicare Part A (hospital insurance), workers and employers contribute equally through a payroll tax of 2.9 percent of earned income. Medicare Part B finances physician care, outpatient, home health, and other services. Enrollment is voluntary, and enrollees are required to pay flat-rate monthly premiums as well as various out-of-pocket fees. Despite premiums and other out-of-pocket payments, the value of benefits received greatly exceeds the value of contributions for most beneficiaries; premiums make up only 24 percent of total expenditures. For example, future benefits have an estimated value of up to six times the lifetime contributions for a retiring couple with one earner (Inglehart 1999b, 328). As a result, virtually everyone eligible enrolls. As Medicare requires patients to pay deductibles (under both Part A and Part B), copayments for physician services (20 percent of the fee above the deductible), and balance billing (any amount a provider opts to extra-bill above the rates paid by Medicare), a large market in "Medigap" insurance has emerged to provide supplementary insurance for these charges.

For its part, Medicaid has become the largest single provider of health insurance in the United States in terms of eligible beneficiaries (Inglehart 1999c, 403). In addition to a range of benefits that receive federally mandated coverage, states have the option to cover additional services such as prescription drugs and dental care under the rubric of Medicaid's matching funding. Despite basic requirements, the discretion of states to set their own standards of eligibility (within federal guidelines) has resulted in large variations in coverage.[4] Inglehart notes, "Indeed, it is no exaggeration to say that there are actually more than 50 Medicaid programs . . . because the rules under which they operate vary so enormously" (1999c, 404).

In 1997 the federal government also devoted new funds for cost-sharing state expansions in health insurance coverage for children under SCHIP (State Children's Health Insurance Program), although total expenditures under this program are not very significant in comparison to total spending under Medicaid. In 2007 with SCHIP legislation set to expire, the Senate passed renewing legislation that would increase SCHIP spending by $35 billion over five years and the House passed a bill that would increase spending by $50 billion over the same period (Pear 2007).

Private employer–provided health insurance is also publicly subsidized through exempting contributions from taxation. These expenditures are roughly one-fifth the magnitude of total public health expenditures, and "if this were a federal health program, it would be the third most expensive one after Medicare and Medicaid" (Inglehart 1999a, 71).[5] Employer-provided health benefits for "extended benefits" (i.e., above and beyond the universal insurance coverage provided in each Canadian province) are similarly subsidized in Canada. Because the range of benefits thus covered is so limited, however, these subsidies are a far less significant element of the federal contribution to health care provision in Canada than in the United States.

Since the inception of ERISA in 1974, U.S. federal and state governments have become more active in regulating the private insurance system. Under ERISA, states are prohibited from regulating private employer–provided insurance by firms that self-insure, which has exempted one-third to one-half of all private insurance on a national basis from state-level regulation. States, however, by virtue of their power to regulate health maintenance organizations (HMOs) and insurance providers, retain the power to regulate the remainder of the private insurance market (National Governors' Association 2000).[6]

The federal Health Insurance Portability and Accountability Act of 1996 (HIPAA) set standards for the segment of the private health insurance market previously protected from state regulation under ERISA and implemented basic federal standards for insurance. In doing so, this legislation provided a basic minimum framework for state regulation of private insurance and introduced nationally uniform regulation of the one-third to one-half of the private insurance market that was previously unregulated (Nichols and Blumberg 1998). HIPAA restricts group plans from discontinuing coverage of individual beneficiaries following job loss, applying eligibility conditions or assessing premiums based on health status and medical history, and excluding individuals plans based on preexisting conditions.[7] HIPAA also mandates guaranteed renewability, ensuring that employers whose employees are covered by a group plan will continue to have access to that coverage. Within these limits, there remains some scope for state variation in regulation of private insurance, discussed below.

Health Care Coverage and Provision in the American States and Canadian Provinces

Within these broad structural frameworks, similarities and differences also are found in the way health services are actually provided. The following section examines these in terms of the broad scope of public intervention; public insurance coverage of the population and services; public regulation of private insurance; and the provision of health services.

Any comparisons between the two countries are complicated by the significant role of the states and provinces in the provision of health care. Within the broad parameters established by the national systems, there is significant variation both among Canadian provinces as well as, more markedly, among American states. There are, of course, also important contrasts between the two countries in these regards. As Banting and Corbett note, "The Canadian system leaves considerable scope for provincial variation; and different provincial approaches to restructuring and expenditure restraint are generating large differences in governance, management, and health service delivery" (2002, 23–24). The result is that "within the broad federal standards, ten discrete provincial health care systems have evolved" (Boase 1996, 24). In turn, Banting and Corbett characterize the U.S. system as bipolar—a common approach to health care provision for the elderly yet with wide subnational variation for the non-elderly. Regarding the latter, state governments have increasingly assumed responsibility for health programs, and state policies have enormous impact on the provision of health insurance in the United States (Rom 1999, 349; Fox and Inglehart 1995, 1).[8]

Public Health Care Coverage and Insurance Regulation

Public health care coverage varies between the two countries but also among states and provinces along two axes—who is covered and what services are covered. While states vary on both axes, variation among Canadian provinces is less significant and limited to services covered.

The Scope of Public Health Care—Expenditures

The claim is often made in Canada that Canadians must be willing to pay higher levels of taxes than their American counterparts in order to support public health care. Similarly, it is widely believed in the United States that the Canadian-style system of health care comes at the cost of significantly higher taxes. Both claims ignore a key point: public expenditures on health care are higher in the United States. To be sure, public expenditures make up a greater proportion of total health expenditures in Canada than the United States; however, total expenditure on health care in the United States significantly exceeds that of Canada (see figure 10.1). Comprising a smaller proportion of a much larger overall total, public health expenditures per capita in the United States came to exceed those in Canada for the first time in 1993 and are now nearly 25 percent higher in the United States than in Canada.

Public Health Insurance Coverage

One of the most oft-noted differences between Canada and the United States is the existence of universal public insurance coverage in Canada, which stands in stark contrast to the significant proportion of the population remaining uninsured and underinsured in the United States. Fully one in five adults under the age of sixty-five in the United States is uninsured while the proportion of children under eighteen years of age is 12 percent (Kaiser Family Foundation 2004).

The proportion of the population that is uninsured varies widely by state.[9] For example, rates of uninsurance range from 5 percent of all children (Hawaii, Massachusetts) to 20 percent of all children (Texas) (see figure 10.2). Thus, depending on the category under examination, some states have more than four times the proportion of uninsured persons than others, and variation among states does not appear to be diminishing. State variations cannot be attributed solely to policy differences; they are also related to cross-state variation in economic conditions and the growth and decline of coverage under employer-sponsored plans. The magnitude of the problem of uninsurance, often perceived in Canadian debates as an inevitable outgrowth of nonuniversal public programs, varies widely.[10]

Figure 10.1   Total Public Health Care Expenditures, U.S. Dollars per Capita, United States and Canada, 1981–2004

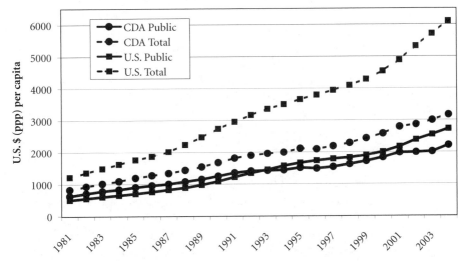

Source: OECD, *Health Expenditure Data, 2006.*

Figure 10.2 Uninsured Children, United States, by State, 2005 (Percentage)

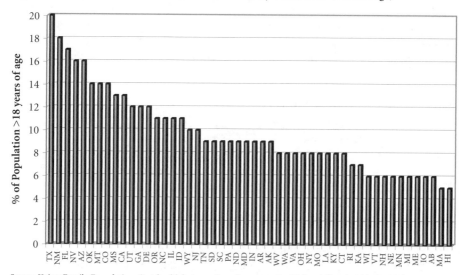

Source: Kaiser Family Foundation, Statehealthfacts.org. http://www.statehealthfacts.kff.org/cgi-bin/healthfacts
.cgi?action = compare&category = Health + Coverage + %26 + Uninsured&subcategory = Insurance + Status &
topic = Distribution + of + Children + 18 + and + Under. Accessed on August 27, 2007.

Cross-state variation in uninsured populations, as noted above, is the result of a variety of factors including public programs for health insurance. As a national program, there is no cross-state variation in persons covered under Medicare. At the same time, there is wide cross-state variation in persons covered under Medicaid, and the resulting coverage rates vary widely. For example, for children under eighteen, Medicaid coverage varies from just under 40 percent in Arkansas, Mississippi, and Vermont to under 15 percent in Nevada (see figure 10.3). Of course, demographic factors are an important factor contributing to this cross-state variation; however, state-level policy differences are also an important factor. In addition to differences in coverage rates, Medicaid expenditures per recipient also vary widely (see figure 10.4). In 2004 Medicaid expenditures per recipient were over three times higher in the highest spending states (Vermont and New York) than those in the lowest spending state (California). As an obvious result of differences in population coverage and expenditure per recipient, total expenditures on Medicaid vary widely by state.

Services Covered by Public Health Insurance

The CHA mandates certain principles for the provision of health insurance in regard to hospital care and physician services, but there are some differences between provinces in services offered under medicare coverage and those outside medicare. While these differences should not be exaggerated, the uniformity of the Canadian system should also not be overstated. The private–public mix varies from

Figure 10.3   Medicaid Coverage, Children Under 18, United States, by State, 2003

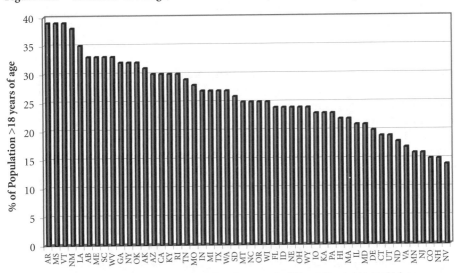

Source: Kaiser Family Foundation, Statehealthfacts.org. http://www.statehealthfacts.kff.org/cgi-bin/healthfacts .cgi?action = compare&category = Health + Coverage + %26 + Uninsured&subcategory = Insurance + Status & topic = Distribution + of + Children + 18 + and + Under. Accessed on August 27, 2007.

Figure 10.4   Medicaid Payments per Enrollee, United States, by State, 2004

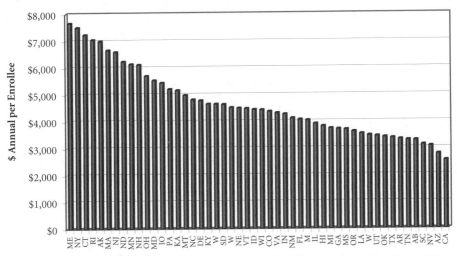

Source: Kaiser Family Foundation, Statehealthfacts.org. http://www.statehealthfacts.org/comparetable.jsp?ind = 183& cat = 4 Accessed on August 27, 2007.

province to province, and this variation seems likely to increase. In areas falling under the strictures of the CHA, there are some differences between provinces. For example, fee differentials for particular services across provinces have reportedly been as high as 50 percent.

Comprehensiveness of coverage varies little between the provinces; what differences there are occur at the margins of a central core of publicly provided health care services. Most of the differences are in pharmacare programs, coverage of health services (dental), alternative health services such as chiropractic services, as well as long-term and home care. Differences in expenditures per capita are notable, being nearly one-third higher in Manitoba than in PEI or Quebec.[11]

While the proportion of total health care funding made up of public funds has been decreasing slightly, there are moderate differences among provinces in the percentage of health care expenditures composed of the public and private sectors. Public sector health expenditures range from 77 percent of total health expenditures in Newfoundland to 66 percent of total health expenditures in Ontario.[12] Passive privatization (the growing significance of those health care sectors that do not have universal public coverage) appears to be the most significant trend in terms of explaining the very moderate decreases in the proportion of public funding across the Canadian health care system (Boychuk and Banting 2008). Differences among provinces in coverage of these areas may presage more significant differences in the ratio of public-to-private spending among provinces.

Both provinces and states vary in providing public drug insurance programs. There is considerable similarity overall between provinces' pharmaceutical coverage and the provision of public drug insurance coverage in the United States: "Canadian drug plans resemble the drug coverage provided in the United States through Medicare and Medicaid. Individuals must meet income, disability, or age criteria to be covered" (Armstrong and Armstrong 1998, 75). Ontario, British Columbia, Saskatchewan, Manitoba, and Québec have "universal" drug insurance programs although, because of high deductibles and copayments, these programs are not very helpful to people other than seniors or those on social assistance. Québec is the one notable exception; it has a universal, although not free at point of service, plan.

All other provinces offer categorical drug insurance programs. In the case of the elderly, the provinces, with only one exception, provide universal coverage that is usually combined with user charges. There is also wide variation among provincial programs in terms of user fees, coverage, and eligibility.[13] Thus it is not surprising that provinces vary widely in their levels of public spending on drugs. Per capita public drug expenditures in high-spending provinces such as Québec ($293.35) are over 80 percent higher than expenditures in provinces such as PEI ($163.37).[14] Provinces also vary widely in the proportion of total drug expenditures that are made up of public expenditures, with public expenditures in Prince Edward Island (23.7 percent) comprising less than a quarter of total drug expenditures while public expenditures in Québec (45.2 percent) make up just under half of total drug expenditures there.

All states make some provision for public drug coverage for low-income families under Medicaid, and thirty states also have programs to provide public insurance for prescription drugs in addition to Medicaid coverage (Kaiser Family Foundation 2005). With the exception of Maine, Maryland, and Wyoming, the states restrict these plans to seniors. Some state programs have very strict income eligibility requirements or restrict coverage in other ways (e.g., specifying for which conditions drug coverage is available). Others, however, such as New York provide relatively broad coverage entailing substantial per recipient costs.

Public drug coverage for seniors in Canada, while similar to that in the United States, historically has been more extensive (in terms of coverage) and more generous (in terms of limited deductibility and copayments). This situation changed significantly, however, with the extension of prescription drug coverage under Medicare in 2006.

Public Regulation of Health Insurance

Prior to HIPAA in 1996, states varied widely in their regulation of privately provided health insurance. Well-worn stories about people losing their insurance coverage, being denied insurance coverage, or facing exorbitant and often unaffordable premiums based on their health or risk category accurately depicted private insurance market conditions in some states. Individual states enacted a variety of regulations, including those mandating community rating (prohibiting the use of age, sex, previous health, and so forth in rate setting), guaranteed issue (mandating that insurers provide all or specific products to any eligible group), guaranteed renewal (prohibiting insurers from refusing to offer insurance to groups or individuals on the basis of past claims), limits on the length of time insurers can deny insurance to individuals with preexisting conditions, and mandatory loss ratios (specifying the ratio of benefits that must be paid out as a proportion of total premiums collected). States varied considerably in the extent to which they used such regulatory tools to intervene in the private health insurance market, ranging from states with virtually no regulation of private insurance to those implementing a considerable range of regulations (Boychuk 2002b).

HIPAA enforced standard regulation of group insurance (including guaranteed issue and renewal as well as limits on use of preexisting conditions in issue and in determining individual rates within the group plan) and individual insurance (including guaranteed issue and renewal). States continue to vary widely in regulating areas ignored by HIPAA. Table 10.1 categorizes states according to the degree to which their regulations cover the three salient types of individual and small-group health insurance regulations not governed by HIPAA. These three categories include "community rating" requirements for both group and individual insurance and limits on preexisting conditions for individual insurance. States range from those with no regulation beyond the federal minimum to those that regulate in every major area left to state discretion (see table 10.1).

States also vary in regard to the role of government in funding and regulating uncompensated care by hospitals, which also plays a significant role in the American system.[15] Medicaid rates and state grants to public hospitals (uncompensated care pools) may help to offset the cost of uncompensated care although these both vary

Table 10.1   Regulation of Individual and Small-group Insurance, United States, by State, 2003

No regulation (0)	Limited regulation (1)	Moderate regulation (2)	Strong regulation (3)
Alabama	California	Connecticut	Maine
Alaska	Colorado	Florida	Massachusetts
Arizona	Georgia	Iowa	New Hampshire
Arkansas	Idaho	Maryland	New Jersey
Delaware	Indiana	Michigan	New Mexico
DC	Kentucky	North Dakota	New York
Hawaii	Louisiana		Oregon
Illinois	Minnesota		Vermont
Kansas	Mississippi		Washington
Missouri	Montana		
Nebraska	Ohio		
Nevada	Rhode Island		
North Carolina	South Carolina		
Oklahoma	South Dakota		
Pennsylvania	Utah		
Tennessee	Virginia		
Texas	Wyoming		
West Virginia			
Wisconsin			

Source: Kaiser Family Foundation, Statehealthfacts.org. Available at www.statehealthfacts.kff.org. Accessed on April 4, 2005.

widely across states. "Although far from perfect, [uncompensated care] has become a standard measure for tracking provision of care for the medically indigent" (Atkinson, Helms and Needleman 1997, 233). The American Hospital Association reports that uncompensated costs equaled 5.5 percent of total hospital costs in 2003 (American Hospital Association 2005).

The public role in funding uncompensated care is closely related to the issue of hospital control, which varies widely among American states. Public hospitals receive state government grants for the provision of uncompensated care while not-for-profit hospitals are expected to provide a minimum level of uncompensated care in order to justify their tax-free status. No similar legal obligation or tax-exempt status applies to private physicians, and as a result, physician services are more difficult to secure for the uninsured.

Provision of Health Services

On the whole, the provision of health services in the two countries is relatively similar. Both systems rely primarily on private, for-profit, fee-for-service physician practice as well as on voluntary, not-for-profit provision of hospital care.

Unlike the situation under Britain's National Health Insurance, in neither the United States nor Canada have physicians generally been salaried government employees. Sometimes surprising to Americans, individuals retain their choice of doctor under the Canadian health care system although this choice is somewhat attenuated in the sense that a patient must get a referral from a general practitioner in order to see a specialist for publicly insured services. The delivery of physician services has been historically quite similar in the two countries, with the exception of the growth in the role of HMOs in the United States from the mid-1970s peaking in the mid-1990s.

Under HMO arrangements, physicians typically either practice through individual practice associations (IPAs) and are remunerated on a capitation (per patient) basis or practice as a salaried physician employed by the plan. HMO enrollment peaked in the mid-1990s (31 percent of total plan enrollment in 1996), and enrollment has declined since then to levels comparable to those of the early 1990s (25 percent of total plan enrollment in 2004) (see figure 10.5). Another important trend over the 1990s has been the displacement of traditional indemnity coverage by PPOs.[16] PPOs preserved the fee-for-service indemnity-type coverage although these organizations are based on a network of providers who have joined the organization by agreeing to accept set fees from the plan that are typically lower than fees that would otherwise be charged. Enrollment in PPOs grew from 11 percent in 1988 to 55 percent in 2004, with a majority of covered American workers now receiving their health benefits under this type of arrangement. Another trend has been the growth in point-of-service (POS) plans, which are usually offered as an indemnity-type option by an HMO and are a hybrid of HMO and PPO arrangements. These plans typically allow full coverage for referrals by the primary-care physician (either within the network or outside) but also allow the individual to self-refer outside the network and still retain partial coverage.

Figure 10.5   Health Plan Enrollment, by Type of Plan, United States, 1988–2004

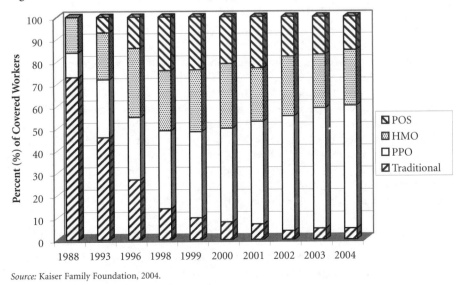

Source: Kaiser Family Foundation, 2004.

The structure of the hospital sector is also similar in the two countries. Both rely predominantly on voluntary not-for-profit hospitals, which make up just over 60 percent of all registered community hospitals in the United States (American Hospital Association 2005) and virtually all hospitals in Canada. State and local government-owned hospitals (which have no analogue in the Canadian health care system) compose just under a quarter of all hospitals. For-profit, investor-owned hospitals—a central element in popular Canadian perception of the U.S. health system—are not a really central element of the U.S. "model." Such hospitals make up only 16 percent of all hospitals in the United States. States vary widely in the mix between these two types of institutions. In Florida, for example, for-profit hospitals make up nearly half of the total while in other states (such as Minnesota, South Dakota, Delaware, Rhode Island, and Vermont) private hospitals do not exist to any significant extent. The mix of hospital control between voluntary not-for-profits and public hospitals (directly owned and controlled by state or local governments) also varies widely across states. In a handful of states, government hospitals constitute over half of all hospitals (and nearly two-thirds in Wyoming). In other states, including South Dakota, Delaware, Rhode Island, and Vermont, both private for-profit and government hospitals are virtually nonexistent; there, voluntary not-for-profits control the entire hospital sector closely in keeping with the Canadian model of hospital control.

The important difference in the way hospitals are funded in the United States vs. Canada is that in the United States hospitals typically receive fee-for-service payments from either public or private insurance providers, and in Canada the hospitals are funded on a global budget basis. Some observers argue that as a result, American voluntary not-for-profit and even public hospitals operate largely as if they were private, for-profit institutions while in Canada, voluntary not-for-profit hospitals operate largely as if they were public institutions.

Conclusions about the Main Differences

The main difference between the two countries in regard to public health insurance is that coverage for hospital and physician services is universal in Canada while comparable public coverage in the United States is limited to those over sixty-five and those with low income. Second, public health insurance in Canada is compulsory in the sense that third-party provision of insurance for publicly covered health services is generally not permitted. This is, of course, not the case in the United States. As a result, even if the structure of health service delivery is roughly similar in the two countries, the funding of health service delivery is quite different. In Canada there is a single-payer system for all publicly insured health services while the U.S. system is much more fragmented, with the existence of multiple payers ranging from public programs, employer-sponsored health insurance plans, health maintenance organizations, and individuals.

Performance of the American and Canadian Health Care Systems

All health care systems attempt to draw a balance between three major goals: quality, access, and cost control. The determination of the appropriate balance between these three goals is a normative value judgment. For any given balance among the three, an important secondary issue is whether the health care system is approaching optimality—that is, whether a higher level of achievement of one goal can still occur without entailing losses on a different value axis. Of course, the outcome of any comparison of the performance of two systems depends on the criteria used, and differential weighting of these criteria will produce markedly different results.

The comparison of the American and Canadian health care systems undertaken below illustrates two points. First, each system performs better than the other in regards to specific criteria—neither system is superior to the other system across the range of criteria. This empirical observation reflects the implicit trade-off between the achievement of the different ends to which a health care system may be aimed. By extension, it also implies that preference for one system over the other is the result of normative value judgment. Second, the differences in the performance of the two systems are clearly related to differences in the structure of the two systems, as outlined above, and do not simply emerge accidentally or as a result of external factors. Rather, they are the direct result of the policy outcomes outlined in the preceding chapters.

Quality

Proponents of the existing system of U.S. health care claim that it delivers health care of the highest quality (while implicitly recognizing necessary trade-offs in terms of costs and access). A good example is President Bush's support during the 2004 presidential debates of the existing system:

> I think government-run health will lead to poor-quality health, will lead to rationing, will lead to less choice. Once a health-care program ends up in a line item in the federal government budget, it leads to more controls. And just look at other countries that have tried to have federally controlled health care. They have poor-quality health care. Our health-care system is the envy of the world because we believe in making sure that the decisions are made by doctors and patients, not by officials in the nation's capital. (Commission on Presidential Debates, 2004)

The following section examines subjective perceptions of health care quality and satisfaction as well as more objective indicators of effectiveness in considering the performance of the American and Canadian health care systems. Subjective perceptions of the quality of care tend to favor the United States, with the exceptions of low-income Americans and sicker adults. At the same time, cross-national differences in perception are not particularly striking. Significant differences in objective outcome measures such as survival rates are also not evident. Important differences between the two countries emerge in timeliness of specialist and surgical care, with the United States performing considerably better than Canada on this score.

Quality and Satisfaction—Subjective Perceptions of Health Care Quality

Interpretations of subjective perceptions of the quality of health care must remain extremely cautious.[17] There is no doubt that whether people perceive themselves to be receiving high-quality health care is an important political consideration. At the same time, public assessments of health care quality are based on popular expectations and perceptions of what "high quality" health care should look like. Differences in perceptions may reveal differences in expectations rather than differences in the objective quality of health care. Noting these caveats, subjective perceptions of health care quality are, with some important caveats, more favorable in the United States than Canada.

Physician perceptions of the quality of care tend to be more favorable among American physicians than their Canadian counterparts. For example, in regard to the quality of hospital care, American physician ratings of the hospitals in which they work are uniformly more favorable (reporting good/excellent) in terms of emergency room facilities (72 percent), nursing staff levels (45 percent), and finding and addressing medical errors (65 percent) than in Canada (51 percent, 30 percent, and 56 percent, respectively) (Blendon et al. 2001, 235). Similarly, hospital administrators in the United States view the quality of U.S. hospitals more favorably than is the case in Canada. The percentage of administrators ranking facilities as very good or excellent was uniformly higher in the United States (intensive care unit 88 percent, operating theaters 81 percent, emergency rooms 57 percent, diagnostic imaging and medical technology 84 percent) than in Canada (intensive care unit 70 percent, operating theaters 62 percent, emergency rooms 33 percent, diagnostic imaging and medical technology 49 percent).

On the other hand, reflecting the unique American experience with managed care, American physicians were significantly more likely to experience limitations on their practice of medicine. Limitations on specialist referrals and diagnostic tests are lower in the United States (27 percent and 21 percent) than in Canada (66 percent and 37 percent); however, they are still reported as a major problem by a significant number of physicians. (These services are limited in Canada primarily by wait times—a topic discussed in more detail below.) Access to hospital care is perceived to be a major problem by a slightly greater proportion of American physicians (38 percent) than Canadian physicians (35 percent). Limitations on drugs that may be prescribed is perceived as a problem by a considerably greater proportion of American (41 percent) than Canadian (17 percent) physicians. Similarly American physicians were much more likely to experience "external review of clinical decisions to control costs" as a major problem in their practice (37 percent) in comparison with Canadian physicians (13 percent). Physicians in both countries were equally likely to feel that "not having enough time with patients" was a major problem for their practice (42 percent).

In keeping with the perceptions of physicians and hospital administrators, recent cross-national surveys suggest that public perceptions of health care quality are also generally more favorable among Americans than is the case for Canadian respondents, with two important caveats. First, favorable perceptions of health service quality vary, unsurprisingly, by health insurance status in the United States and are lower among the minority of the population who are uninsured. Second, among sicker adults, American respondents tend to be less satisfied with the health services they have received than sicker adults in Canada (discussed more fully in the following section).

Substantial majorities of respondents in both countries perceived the quality of health services they received to be good or excellent (see figure 10.6). Insured Americans were slightly more likely than Canadians to perceive their health services they received as excellent while uninsured Americans were significantly less likely than Canadians to perceive the health services they received as excellent. An inverse pattern holds for the proportion of respondents in each group perceiving health services as only fair or poor. Differences among Canadians and insured Americans are even less notable for physician services. The perceived quality of physician services was virtually identical among Canadians and insured Americans, although it was lower among the U.S. uninsured (see figure 10.7).

Perceptions of the quality of care also vary by income status in both countries as well as by insurance status in the United States. Perceptions of the quality of health care services in Canada vary significantly based on income.[18] While both above-average income and below-average income Canadian respondents tended to view the quality of care they received favorably (60 percent and 51 percent, respectively, rating it as excellent or very good), individuals with below-average income were two-thirds more likely (15 percent) to perceive services to be of a fair/poor quality than those with above-average incomes (9 percent).

Differences based on income were even more pronounced in the United States (including among insured Americans) and heavily condition conclusions that can be drawn on the basis of insurance status alone. American respondents with above-average incomes (65 percent) were more likely to perceive care to be of excellent

Figure 10.6 Perceived Quality of Health Services, United States and Canada, 2002–03

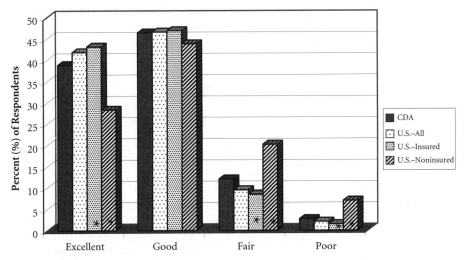

Statistically significant
Source: United States National Center for Health Statistics, Center for Disease Control and Statistics Canada, *Joint Canada/United States Survey of Health, 2002–03.*

Figure 10.7   Perceived Quality of Physician Services, United States and Canada, 2002–03

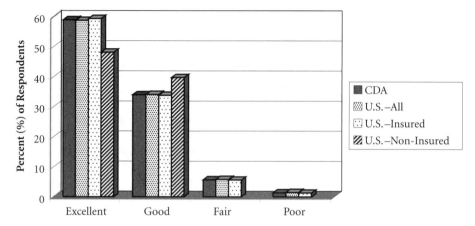

Source: United States National Center for Health Statistics, Center for Disease Control and Statistics Canada, *Joint Canada/United States Survey of Health, 2002–03.*
Notes:"Fair" and "poor" responses for U.S. non-insured not reported due to low sample size and variability.

or very high quality than those with below-average incomes (45 percent)—with Canadians of both above- and below-average income falling between.[19] The inverse holds for perceptions of fair- or poor-quality care. American respondents with below-average income and no insurance coverage are much more likely (28 percent) to experience fair/poor care than those with insurance coverage. Insured respondents with below-average income are still considerably more likely (17 percent) to perceive fair/poor than insured respondents with above-average income (7 percent). Canadian respondents with both below- and above-average income fell between these two groups of insured Americans, with 15 percent and 9 percent, respectively, experiencing fair/poor care.

Effectiveness—Objective Measures of Health Care Quality

There has been a broad movement across western industrialized countries in general toward the objective measurement of health care quality and performance indicators.[20] The following section considers three broad classes of indicators—process indicators, avoidable events, and survival rates. Neither system is demonstrably superior to the other across these objective measures of outcomes.

On process indicators such as cancer screening rates and immunizations, there is little discernable difference between the two countries on any of the individual outcome indicators (see table 10.2). In terms of avoidable events, such as the incidence of pertussis, measles, and hepatitis, the United States fares better than Canada although even here the picture is mixed, with the United States performing significantly better on two indicators and significantly worse on one.[21]

Table 10.2 **Comparable Health Performance Indicators, United States and Canada, 2002**

Class	Indicator	Canada	U.S.	Comparison
Process	Breast cancer screening rate (%)	73	70	Comparable
	Cervical cancer screening (%)	77	77	Comparable
	Influenza vaccination rate, age 65 + (%)	67	66	Comparable
	Polio vaccination rate, age 2 (%)	87	90	Comparable
Avoidable events	Pertussis (per 100,000)	20.0	2.7	U.S. better
	Measles (per 100,000)	0.1	0.04	U.S. better
	Hepatitis B (per 100,000)	4.2	6.3	Canada better
Survival rates	Breast cancer survival rate (%)	78	86	U.S. better
	Cervical cancer survival rate (%)	74	75	Comparable
	Colorectal cancer survival rate (%)	60	58	Comparable
	Child leukemia survival rate (%)	81	76	Canada better
	Non-Hodgkin's lymphoma survival rate (%)	62	63	Comparable
	Kidney transplant survival rate (%)	94	83	Canada better
	Liver transplant survival rates (%)	87	73	Canada better

Both the process indicators and avoidable events have a strong public health element to them, and it is to indicators such as survival rates where popular perceptions regarding the quality of the health care system proper would turn. Comparisons of U.S. and Canadian survival rates for various categories of medical condition reveal a picture of rough comparability.[22] Comparisons of survival rates for five different types of cancer suggest a rough parity between the United States and Canada, with the former having superior performance in survival rates for breast cancer but inferior performance for child leukemia and comparable rates on the three remaining types of cancer. Canada performs markedly better in terms of organ-transfer survival rates although this may be primarily because the Canadian public health care system ensures that such transplants occur in those cases with the greatest chances of success.

Quality—Timeliness of Health Service Provision

The set of objective performance indicators outlined above are very broad indicators of health system performance. They obviously leave out significant elements of health system performance—especially quality-of-life indicators that are much more difficult to measure. For example, long waiting times for various health services (especially in cases that are nonemergency or not life-threatening) may have important impacts on quality of life but not necessarily show up in data on avoidable events or survival rates. Such considerations are an especially important concern in Canada where long waiting times have raised important questions about the overall performance of the health care system.

PRIMARY CARE

Little difference is found between the two countries in terms of access to primary care. Canada does have a larger supply on a per capita basis of basic resources central to primary care, such as general practitioners, nurses, and hospital beds. Canada has 25 percent more practicing general practice physicians, 22 percent more practicing nurses, and 10 percent more available acute-care hospital beds per capita than the United States (Organization for Economic Cooperation and Development [OECD] 2006). In terms of perceptions of the timeliness of access to primary care, the differences between the United States and Canada are limited. There is no difference between the two countries in the proportion of respondents unable to get a same-day appointment (65 percent in Canada, 64 percent in the United States) or difficulty in getting primary care on evenings or weekends (41 percent in both the United States and Canada). However, somewhat more respondents reported emergency waiting times as a "big problem" in Canada (37 percent) than in the United States (31 percent). Emergency department problems such as "critical-care bypass" in Canada (where emergency patients are diverted to a nearby hospital) also exist in the United States, where just under 70 percent of all urban hospitals reported in 2004 having spent some time on "emergency department diversion" (American Hospital Association 2005).

SPECIALIST CARE AND ELECTIVE SURGERY

Differences in regard to access to specialist care, nonemergency surgery, and high-tech diagnostic equipment are significantly starker. Of physicians surveyed, a much higher percentage of physicians in Canada responded that "limitations or long waits for specialist referrals" and "long wait times for surgical or hospital care" were a major problem for their practice in Canada (66 percent and 64 percent respectively) than in the United States (27 percent and 7 percent respectively.). Physicians in Canada were also more likely to experience "limitations in ordering diagnostic test or procedures" (37 percent) in comparison with their American counterparts (21 percent)—presumably because of waiting times resulting from a lower supply of high-technology diagnostics. Physicians in both countries were equally predisposed (35 percent in Canada, 38 percent in the United States) to respond that "limitations on hospital care" were a major problem (Blendon et al. 2001).

In terms of supply, there are 1.4 specialists per 1,000 population in the United States in comparison with 1.1 in Canada. Given the difference in the density of general practitioners, the ratio of specialists to general practitioners in the United States is 1.75 to 1 while in Canada the ratio is 1.1 to 1 (OECD 2006). The health care system in the United States is significantly more geared toward specialist care than is the case in Canada, where the health care system rests more heavily on care provided by general practitioners. As for access to medical technology, the United States has more than three times as many magnetic resonance imagers (MRI) as Canada, more than seven times as many lithotripters, and just under 40 percent more computer tomography scanners (CT scans) on a per capita basis (OECD 2006).[23]

Among "sicker adults,"[24] just over half of Canadian respondents reported that it was somewhat or very difficult to see a specialist (53 percent) while the proportion of American respondents reporting problems seeing a specialist was 39 percent. More than one-third of American respondents (37 percent) had to wait more than one month for surgery. In Canada this figure was nearly double (63 percent). Furthermore, more than one-quarter of Canadian respondents (27 percent) waited more than four months for nonemergency surgery—more than five times the proportion of respondents in the United States (5 percent) who waited a similar length of time.

Waiting times in Canada vary significantly by type of procedure (Esmail and Walker 2004). Waiting times (from referral by GP to treatment) range from six to eight weeks for medical and radiation oncology to thirty-eight weeks for orthopedic surgery such as hip and knee replacements and tend to vary by the urgency of the procedure. For example, patients needing urgent cardiovascular surgery experience a median wait time of roughly ten days (after an appointment with a specialist) while patients undergoing elective cardiovascular surgery experience median wait times of just under seven weeks. A second striking trend is that waiting times for all categories of procedure (except elective cardiovascular surgery) have increased significantly over the past decade—with wait times for some procedures such as orthopedic surgery and plastic surgery more than doubling (Esmail and Walker 2004, 32).

Similarly, there are significant waiting times for access to high-technology diagnostic equipment such as CT scans (average waiting time of 5.2 weeks), MRIs (average national waiting time of 12.6 weeks), and ultrasound (average national waiting time of 3.1 weeks) (Romanow 2002, 140–41). Waiting times vary on a province-by-province basis—albeit less widely for CT scans and ultrasounds than for MRIs. In regard to MRIs, the average wait time in Newfoundland of 33.5 weeks is nearly three times the national average and more than five and one-half times the shortest provincial average (in neighboring Prince Edward Island).

Access

Access to health care—the ability to get needed health care services—is less problematic in Canada than in the United States. If one of the main barriers to access to public health services in Canada is waiting times, the main barrier to access to health services in the United States is cost, and as a result, access varies significantly by insurance status.

Access—Unmet Health Care Needs

In terms of physicians' perceptions of access, Canadian physicians are much less likely (12 percent) than their American counterparts (17 percent) to think that it is "often" the case that patients get sicker because they cannot get the health care they need (Blendon et al. 2001, 238). Similarly, Canadian physicians (24 percent) are less likely than their American counterparts (36 percent) to think that it is "often" the case that patients do not receive preventive care (Blendon et al. 2001, 238). The proportion of physicians reporting that it is "often" the case that patients lack access to the newest drugs or medical technology is the same in both countries (26 percent).

These physician perceptions fit with the reported incidence of unmet health care needs among survey respondents. There is no statistically significant difference in the incidence of unmet health care needs between Canadian respondents (10.7 percent) and insured American respondents (10.3 percent). At the same time, uninsured American respondents are far more likely to experience unmet health care needs (40 percent) (Statistics Canada 2004).

The incidence of unmet health care needs varies both within Canada and the United States with age and income; however, in both cases, the variation is greater in the United States (Statistics Canada 2004). The prevalence of unmet health care needs among adults aged eighteen to forty-four years is higher in the United States (15.8 percent) than in Canada (12.2 percent). Conversely the incidence of unmet health care needs in the United States is lower (6.5 percent) than Canada (7.4 percent) for those over sixty-five years of age (although this difference is not statistically significant).

The incidence of unmet health care needs also varies widely in both countries based on income, and again, this variation is wider in the United States than Canada (Statistics Canada 2004). In the latter, for example, the middle-income quintile is twice less likely (7.9 percent) to experience unmet health care needs than the bottom-income quintile (17.4 percent). In the United States, the bottom quintile (26.6 percent) is nearly three times more likely than the middle-income quintile (9.3 percent) to experience unmet health care needs. The differences between the two countries in unmet health care needs by quintile is statistically insignificant except for the bottom quintile, where the rate in the United States (26.6 percent) is more than 50 percent higher than the rate in Canada (17.4 percent).

Access Problems from Cost and Insurance Coverage

While 54 percent of sicker adults in Canada listed doctor and bed shortages as a major problem with the health care system and 27 percent listed wait times (5 percent and 3 percent in the United States, respectively), the main problems in the United States with the health care system, according to sicker adults, were high costs (48 percent) and inadequate insurance coverage (25 percent)—13 percent and 8 percent, respectively, in Canada. A much higher proportion of respondents in the United States did not receive various health services because cost. Sicker Americans are much more likely than sicker Canadians to respond that they did not get a service because of costs: 28 percent compared with 9 percent in Canada for medical care in general, 26 percent compared with 10 percent for tests or treatments, 35 percent compared with 19 percent for prescriptions, and 40 percent compared with 35 percent for dental care (Blendon et al. 2003).

These differences are consistent with differences in perceptions among American and Canadian physicians of the barriers to access posed by cost (Blendon et al. 2001, 236). American physicians (52 percent) are much more likely than their Canadian counterparts (32 percent) to be "very concerned" that patients cannot afford the care they need. They are more than three times more likely to respond that their patients "often" have difficulty affording out-of-pocket costs (61 percent) than their Canadian counterparts (19 percent). Physicians in the United States are more pre-disposed to experience patients not being able to "afford necessary prescription drugs" (48 percent) as a major problem for their practice than Canadian physicians (17 percent).

The problem is not simply, as one might presume, a function of higher out-of-pocket costs in the United States. Out-of-pocket payments for health services were substantial in both countries and comprise a slightly higher percentage of total health care expenditures in Canada than in the United States (see table 10.3). While these payments were higher in the United States ($690 per capita in 2000) in com-parison with Canada ($490 per capita in U.S. dollars using purchasing power parity) in dollar terms, as a percentage of total household consumption, they were compa-rable in the two countries: 2.9 percent in the United States and 2.7 percent in Canada (Huber and Orosz 2003, 15). At issue in explaining the higher prevalence of unmet health care needs in the United States is the distribution of these costs.

On every measure, uninsured Americans experience the most severe access prob-lems (see fig. 10.8). More than half of uninsured respondents experienced difficulties getting specialty care, did not get tests, treatments, follow-up, or prescriptions because of costs, and have problems paying their medical bills. There is important variation in access even among Americans with health insurance depending on income. Whether insured Americans experienced less difficulty than Canadians in receiving specialty care depends on whether they are above or below average income. The proportion of respondents not receiving a test, treatment, or follow-up care because of cost was higher, even for insured Americans with above-average income, than for any Canadian respondents—including those with below-average income. Even for insured Americans with above-average income, one in ten respondents had problems paying their medical bills. In Canada, the experience of this problem by poll respondents is dependent on their income—with below-average-income Canadian respondents experiencing this problem to a greater degree than above-average-income insured Americans and above-average-income Canadians experiencing this problem to a much lesser degree.

Table 10.3 Out-of-pocket Health Expenditures, United States and Canada, 2000

	% of total health expenditures[a]	$ per capita (US ppp)[a]	% of total household consumption[b]
United States	15.2	$690	2.9
Canada	15.8	$490	2.7

[a] OECD, 2003
[b] Huber and Orosz, 2003.

Figure 10.8   Access Problems Due to Cost, by Income and Insurance Status, United States and Canada, 2001

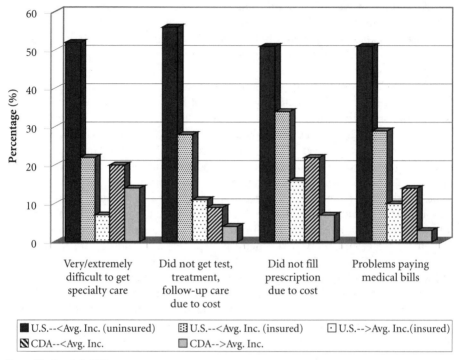

Source: Blendon et al., 2002.

Satisfaction—Quality, Timeliness, Access

Satisfaction with health services is a much broader measure of perceptions than those outlined above in terms of both the breadth of the term "satisfaction" (presumably incorporating, for most respondents, various factors including quality, timeliness, and access) as well as the breadth implied by "health services" presumably including, for most respondents, both hospital and physician care as well as primary and specialist care.

In comparison with insured Americans (54.7 percent), Canadians are less likely to be "very satisfied" (43.7 percent) and more likely (43.3 percent) than insured Americans (36.5 percent) to simply be "satisfied" (Statistics Canada 2004) Differences between the two groups in levels of dissatisfaction are statistically significant although this group makes up a small majority of all respondents in both cases with 5.5 percent (Canada) and 4.2 percent (U.S.) of respondents being "dissatisfied" and 2.6 percent (Canada) and 1.3 percent (U.S.) of respondents being "very dissatisfied." Although satisfaction rates of uninsured Americans are surprisingly high (38.9 percent being very satisfied and 40.4 percent being satisfied), uninsured Americans are much more likely (9.1 percent) to be "very dissatisfied" with health services received than either insured Americans or Canadians. In terms of satisfaction with physician services, insured Americans are slightly more likely to be "very satisfied" than Canadians (67.8 percent versus 64.2 percent) and less likely to be "very dissatisfied" (1.7 percent versus 3.6 percent). Again, uninsured Americans are much less likely than Canadians to be "very satisfied" (51.5 percent) and much more likely to be "very dissatisfied" (18.2 percent).

Nevertheless, among sicker adults, American respondents tended to be less satisfied with the overall health system than Canadian respondents.[25] Sicker respondents in the United States are less likely to be very satisfied (18 percent in the United States, 21 percent in Canada) or fairly satisfied (36 percent in the United States, 41 percent in Canada.) They are more likely to be not very satisfied (25 percent in the United States, 23 percent in Canada) or not at all satisfied (19 percent in the United States, 13 percent in Canada) with the health services they received.

Overall Cost and Cost Containment

Both public expenditures on health care as well as overall health care costs have been growing more rapidly in the United States than in Canada since the early 1970s. There are a variety of drivers of overall expenditure increases, including growth and change in the health services supplied. However, there are two elements that are key to higher overall costs in the United States relative to those in Canada— higher and more rapidly growing administrative costs and medical inflation.

Administrative Costs

Administrative costs are higher in the United States as a result of the multi-payer system by which health care providers must determine who and how much to bill as well as incur the administrative costs associated with payment collection. In the Canadian system, health care providers (for those services covered under public insurance) deal with only one payer—the provincial public health insurance program.

As a result, administrative costs are considerably higher in the United States although just how much higher is a matter of some dispute. Woolhandler, Campbell, and Himmelstein (2003) estimate that the cost of health care administration in the United States in 1999 was $1,059 per capita and $307 in Canada (in U.S. dollars)—31 percent of total health care spending in the United States and 16.7 percent in Canada.

It is not simply that the American system generates a higher level of administrative costs in proportion to costs in Canada but, rather, that administrative costs in the United States have been growing much more rapidly. For example, the percentage of the health care labor force made up by administrative personnel in the United States increased by over 50 percent from 1969 (18.2 percent) to 1999 (27.3 percent).[26] The Organization for Economic Cooperation and Development (OECD) calculated the total expenditures for health administration and insurance in the United States at just over double expenditures in Canada in 1960. By 2001 this ratio was nearly six to one (OECD 2006).

Medical Inflation

On balance, the single-payer system appears better placed to restrain growth in relative prices of health care although there is debate as to the degree to which single-payer systems necessarily have lower rates of growth in medical costs (Thorpe 1994). In a single-payer system, health care providers negotiate directly with the single government insurance plan in regards to fee increases providing a robust mechanism of cost control relative to multiple payer systems. Similarly, hospital costs in Canada are set by global budgets, which provides a much stronger mechanism of cost control in contrast to the United States.

Between 1991 and 2001, price increases for total medical expenditures were 17.3 percent in Canada and just over 40 percent in the United States (see table 10.4). In the Canadian case, inflation for medical services has generally kept pace with general inflation in the Canadian economy; however, in the U.S. case, the price of medical services increased by over 15 percent relative to all goods and services (e.g., over and above general inflation in the economy). Regardless of the theoretical debates as to whether single-payer systems are necessarily more effective at cost control than multiple-payer systems, the Canadian health care system has been much more successful in practice at restraining medical inflation than the U.S. system.

Performance

In terms of subjective judgments of the quality of the two systems, Americans have more positive perceptions of the quality of health services. However, this overall conclusion is conditioned by the exceptions of the uninsured, those with below-average income, and sicker adults. These differences in perception are not, however, evident in objective outcome measures. Thus, comparisons of quality must be cautious and overall conclusions subject to numerous caveats.

There are, however, a set of starker conclusions that can be drawn. In terms of quality, the main difference between the two systems is the poor performance of the Canadian system in providing timely access to specialist and surgical care. In

Table 10.4   Price Indices for Health Expenditures, United States and Canada, 1991–2001

1991 to 2001	Total expenditures on health		Total expenditures on pharmaceutical (and medical nondurables)		Private consumption on health	
	% change in price index	% change in relative price index (GDP)	% change in price index	% change in relative price index (GDP)	% change in price index	% change in relative price index (GDP)
Canada	+ 17.3	+ 0.8	+ 16.9	+ 0.6	+ 22.1	+ 5.2
United States	+ 40.6	+ 15.0	+ 40.5	+ 15.0	+ 42.3	+ 16.5

Source: OECD, 2003.

terms of access, the experience of unmet health care needs is more significant in the United States, where cost acts as a major barrier to access and the receipt of health services is much more sharply stratified by both income and insurance status. In terms of cost control, the Canadian system has performed significantly better than the American system. The overall conclusions that could be drawn regarding the superiority of either system depends on the weight that is placed on each of these assessment criteria.

Conclusions

As outlined above, the systems of public health insurance in the United States and Canada demonstrate important differences but, also, important similarities. These particular patterns of similarity and difference between the two systems are strongly in keeping with the interpretation of the historical developments of these systems outlined above: the two systems started from roughly equivalent starting points and then proceeded through a serpentine process of historical development in which each was strongly conditioned by unique historical circumstances—with some similarities becoming embedded while, at the same time, important differences emerged. As a result of this process of development, the systems that emerged in both cases are considerably more complex than if either were a more straightforward projection of national political culture or institutional configuration, and neither is an archetype—or necessarily even a good example—of the "model" that supposedly underpins each. The differences in health system performance outlined in the section above clearly reflect the structure of the health care system in each country and the place of public health insurance within that larger structure. In doing so, these differences in performance also reflect the long-term effects of the politics of race in the United States and the politics of territorial integration in Canada on the provision of public health insurance in each of these countries.

CHAPTER ELEVEN

Conclusions and Implications

HEALTH CARE REFORM remains a critical political issue in both the United States and Canada. What does the reinterpretation of the historical development of public health insurance suggest about current efforts at reform, their likely direction, and their chances of success? In answering these questions, this chapter briefly recapitulates the alternative interpretation of the development of public health insurance in the United States and Canada. It then briefly considers the theoretical and conceptual implications of this reinterpretation. Finally, it considers the policy implications of this alternative explanation for current debates regarding health care reform in both countries.

The differences that emerged as public health insurance developed in the two countries were rooted in the distinctive societal characteristics of the nations in which they evolved, the interaction of these characteristics with other factors, and the way the nature of these interactions have shifted. Because these central causal dynamics and the relationships among them were not fixed nor was it the case that the outcomes resulted from the unfolding of a relatively deterministic linear sequence, prospects for reform—and possibly shifts in existing paths—are likely more open than other interpretations might suggest. In the United States, the role of race in the politics of health care has shifted, which may, along with a number of other factors outlined in chapter 5, open up new possibilities for reform. At the same time, race remains an important latent factor that, if energized, could even more seriously complicate efforts at national health insurance reform than in the Clinton reform era. In Canada territorial politics remain central to the politics of public health insurance, and tensions along this axis will undoubtedly shape health care reforms, possibly in new directions.

The Politics of Race and Territorial Integration
in the United States and Canada

The development of health insurance in Canada provides a comparative perspective on the exceptional pattern of development in the United States. The comparison casts doubt on interpretations that explain the lack of national public health insurance in the United States by placing causal preeminence on American political culture, American institutions and its system of federalism, and, as in the now conventional path-dependence arguments, the scope of private benefits. At the same time, much as the politics of health reform in the United States became embroiled in the politics of civil rights, the Canadian example illustrates the degree to which the politics of national health insurance reform were intertwined with broader political processes—in Canada, national territorial integration.

The Politics of Race in the United States

The politics of race were central in the history of public health insurance in the United States. The failure to include national health insurance in the New Deal pushed federal health insurance reform into a period where it became deeply entangled with the issue of civil rights. As the federal government became more clearly committed to desegregation after 1945, federal intervention in virtually any policy area could be construed as a potential challenge to the racial status quo, and the specific federal approach to health insurance reform in this period exacerbated these fears. In this context progress on national public health insurance met powerful resistance. After a relatively short period in which comprehensive public health insurance was considered, federal policymakers quickly realized that some sort of compromise was required. Providing public health insurance to the aged through Social Security would result in a more limited program—thus generating less resistance—and would symbolically re-create the compromises of the New Deal. Medicaid, added at the last minute to mute opposition to the central plank of health insurance reform (Medicare), reprised another compromise of the New Deal—leaving determinations of eligibility and scope of services covered for needs-based insurance to the states. Adding Medicaid also effectively excluded important areas of health service provision, such as nursing home care, from the full application of civil rights requirements. Compromises over hospital and doctor remuneration, resulting from the need to ensure smooth take off given the imperatives of racial desegregation of health services, resulted in the very high costs of the Medicare/Medicaid programs and, in turn, significantly constrained future reforms. As a result, efforts at broader public health insurance expansion were pushed into a period much less propitious for reform.

Race was a central element of the period in which American public health insurance policy was initially formed and helps to explain the lack of national public health insurance as well as the specific structure of the programs that did emerge. In this way the politics of race has had a crucial legacy for the politics of health care reform today. While race still plays a role in health care politics in the United States, its role has shifted, and it does not have the same direct impact on health insurance reform it did from the mid-1940s through the mid-1960s. Public programs helped break the back of segregated health services in the late 1960s and early 1970s. Since then, they have contributed to shifting public perceptions of the uninsured—as well as dulling the racial identification of programs such as Medicaid—by folding in coverage for minority groups with white, middle-class recipients. As a result of these shifts, the role of race in shaping public health care debates in the Clinton era was transformed but was, nonetheless, crucial in shaping the outcomes of the debates—especially in shaping the interaction between health care reform and such major areas of reform as crime control and welfare reform. The intersection between the politics of race and the politics of health reform helps explain why health reform shared company with these two other policy planks, why it proceeded as far as it did, and ultimately, why it failed. In the Clinton years, race did not represent the same type of immediate structural barrier to reform that it once did, but it was a powerful latent issue in shaping and limiting the possibilities for health care reform.

Health Care as Statecraft: Territorial Politics in the Canadian Federation

Social policies—and public health insurance especially—have played a central role in the politics of territorial integration in Canada and, in turn, have themselves been deeply and indelibly marked by territorial politics, though with varying effects. At times territorial politics frustrated expansionary reforms. At other times it drove them.

Initial proposals for public health insurance reform at the national level in Canada were considerably more comprehensive (in the scope of services covered) and more nationally uniform than the reforms that would be eventually adopted in a halting process starting a decade later and culminating nearly three decades later. Deep tensions between the federal and provincial levels of government—most notably Québec—over control of this tool of state-building foreclosed these early reform options. The division of powers in Canada acted as the institutional equivalent of the separation of powers in the United States. In both cases, divided interests defeated national health insurance plans that threatened to encroach on established social relations. The timing of the initial failure of national health insurance proposals meant that when public health insurance finally emerged in Canada, it did not enjoy strong political support from key federal and provincial leaders and it faced the opposition of the medical profession. Ultimately this resulted in a more piecemeal approach to reform and limited universal public health insurance coverage to hospital care—and, later, medical care—insurance.

In fact, had it not been for a series of fortuitous events, public health insurance on a national basis might not have emerged at all. The first of these events was the provincial government in Saskatchewan committing to implement a hospital insurance scheme before realizing that federal cost-sharing would not be forthcoming—a misperception that created a window of opportunity in which the constraining effects of federalism were suspended. A national program only emerged a decade later, largely as the result of jockeying between the federal government and the government of Ontario as each blamed the other for the failure to implement a hospital insurance program. Any number of changes in circumstance might have prevented the development of a federal cost-sharing program for hospital insurance. Had this been the case, the Saskatchewan government certainly would not have had the financial wherewithal to proceed with physician care insurance, which it did and which helped set the stage for the next round of national-level reform.

When Saskatchewan proceeded with physician care insurance in the 1960s, prospects for the adoption of a federal program looked dim. The balance was tipped in favor of reform as public physician care insurance offered the federal government a crucial strategic opportunity to create a link with individual citizens—most important, in Québec—on a pan-Canadian basis. Similarly, fifteen years later, in the absence of any provincial prodding and little cabinet or caucus support, the federal Liberal government signaled its intention, in the crucial weeks leading up to the Québec referendum, to reinforce national principles bringing the provision of public health insurance up to the standards available inside Québec, thereby allowing the federal government to stake its claim as the sole guarantor of the right of Canadian citizens to universal, comprehensive, first-dollar, public coverage for hospital and physician care insurance. Over the twenty years since the adoption of the CHA, the centrality of health care to territorial politics and vice versa has become increasingly evident. Health care displaced constitutional issues to become the single most important focus of federal–provincial relations in Canada.

The federal government, following the Québec referendum of 1995, struggled to reassert its role in health care. This development followed a much older pattern of health care initiatives at the federal level following flare-ups of nationalist sentiment in Québec. The first public commitment at the federal level to national health insurance (undertaken by the Liberal Party in 1919) occurred in the context of a serious disruption in relations between Québec and the rest of Canada—encapsulated most notably in the first conscription crisis of 1917. National health insurance reemerged on the federal political agenda with the federal announcement of a national health insurance plan in the same year as the second Québec conscription crisis in 1942. Proposals for a federal Medicare program resurfaced in the context of the Quiet Revolution in the 1960s. The federal government renewed its commitment to vigorous enforcement of national principles through the CHA in the context of the 1980 Québec referendum. Finally, in the immediate wake of the 1995 Québec referendum, the federal government again began a decade-long effort to renew its role in the health care field—the final outcome of which has not yet been decisively determined.

Implications for Understanding Public Health Insurance

The interpretation presented here has implications for how we study public policy—both in terms of policy understanding and in terms of policy learning. Most critically, this interpretation emphasizes the need to be attuned to the effects of conjunctures between large-scale processes of development and developments within particular policy fields. Second, it urges caution in attempting to apply policy lessons from one national context to another.

Historical Institutionalism and Path Dependence

The interpretation offered here serves to highlight the problematic nature of a number of more general trends in North American policy analysis: a predilection to explain policy development within an isolated national context (a characteristic that is especially evident in the study of public health insurance in both the United States and Canada); a tendency to compartmentalize policy arenas and abstract them from their complex linkages with both other policy areas and broader political issues; and finally, concomitant with the rise of historical institutionalism as a framework for historical policy analysis, a predisposition to be unduly institutionalist (focusing too narrowly on institutions or institutionalized path dependence) while being insufficiently historical—paying too little attention to the historical and social contexts in which policies developed. In arguing that racial and territorial politics were crucial in the development of distinctive approaches to health care in the two countries, an important central point is that, although political culture, institutions, path dependence, and historical sequence all played important roles in shaping the development of health care in each country, the emergence of differences in the health care systems was ultimately rooted in the structure and nature of the two societies.

While positive feedback mechanisms associated with path dependence are evident at important points in the development of public health insurance in each country, conjunctures between the development of public health insurance and other large-scale processes unfolding simultaneously—especially the extension of civil rights in the United States and the process of nation-building in Canada—were critical in shaping the path of public health insurance. The sequence of events—the timing and stage of each of these processes when they intersected—was also critical in determining their impact on the development of public health insurance in each country.

Policy Learning and the "American" and "Canadian" Models of Public Health Insurance

Given the values that are portrayed in contemporary debates as underpinning the Canadian health care system, one would expect to find a system much more like the one initially contemplated in the early 1940s—a much more comprehensive system of public health insurance operated on a truly national basis by the federal government. Given historical circumstances and political reality, however, this was not to be. On the other hand, the system that developed in the United States is hardly the epitome of rugged individualism or the relatively unfettered reign of market forces—a point that contemporary critics of the Medicare system often emphasize. One observer has recently referred to the U.S. health insurance system as "quasi-socialistic" (Pipes 2004). Despite being obviously overblown, such claims highlight the considerable dissonance between the extent of public intervention in the health care system in practice and the free market philosophical underpinnings of the system as most citizens—and even the outgoing president—perceive them.

As a result of the very particular trajectories of health insurance development, the use in either country of the example of health insurance in the other is often more appropriate for policy understanding as opposed to direct policy learning, which must be undertaken with much greater caution. Despite the prevalence of claims in Canada, the challenges facing the American system are not endemic to a

mixed system of public and private health care but result from the system developing at a time when race was central in U.S. politics. Similarly, the contemporary
stresses on the Canadian health care system are not inherent in universal public
health insurance but result from the development of this system in the particular
context of Canadian federalism that has, in the recent past, overemphasized the
financial strains of health care provision, created an impression of crisis that is not
accurate, and stymied most recent efforts at reform (see Boychuk 2002a, 2002b,
2003, 2004b, 2007a).

Implications for Health Care Reform

This reinterpretation of the history of public health insurance development has
specific implications for reform in both countries. Of course, any consideration of
reform must begin with a caveat highlighting the need for caution and the tenuous
nature of prognostications. Nevertheless, this historical interpretation offers possible outlines of development.

Public Health Insurance, National Values, and Political Institutions

The differences in health care provision in the United States and Canada are not
the natural extension of distinctive national political values or political institutions.
While rhetorically powerful, such claims do not represent a historically grounded
understanding of the development of public health insurance in the two countries.

As argued in this book, public health insurance in Canada contributed to shaping
popular values related to public health care programs rather than arising out of
those values. Second, while it is the case that there are "some policies that national
values rule out," "a wide variety of social institutions can be consistent with the
same set of values," and as a result, "significant reforms might be undertaken without threatening national values" (Marmor, Okma, and Latham 2002, iv). The broad
history of public health insurance reform in these two countries is clearly suggestive
of this—both countries entertained a range of reform options that largely over-
lapped. This overlap, the similar tenor and language of debates in the two countries,
and broad similarities in public opinion have long suggested that the values underpinning the model of each country do not lie outside the boundaries posed by the
public value consensus in the other country.

Illustrations of the ability of public programs to shape public opinion stretch
well back into the development of public health insurance in Canada. As outlined
in chapter 7, the highly controversial universal medical care plan in Saskatchewan
quickly came to have widespread public acceptance—protecting it from dismantle-
ment even after a change to a governing party hostile to universal public insurance.
At the federal level central design characteristics of early public health insurance
programs such as universality and the phasing out of coinsurance and premiums,
which were simply artifacts of the imperatives of federal–provincial cost-sharing,
later came to have impressive resonance in the Canadian public psyche and contributed to the redefinition of public health insurance as a right of citizenship. At the

same time, it is crucial to recognize that early health insurance proposals in the United States often challenged public opinion on accepted social practices—such as segregation in the South—that was much more intransigent than public opinion on the issue of health insurance per se and likely much more intransigent than public opinions on health care today.

Given that the specific designs of public health insurance systems in the two countries were shaped primarily by forces other than cultural values, the cultural values that the public and policymakers now choose to see reflected in these programs lie in the eye of the beholder. They are not a historical inheritance passed down through these programs or a natural state of being to which future reforms must conform. While the differences between these two systems may now be relatively well embedded, the institutional and political supports for them were politically constructed and, as such, can be deconstructed or reconstructed.

In the debates over health care reform in the early 1990s, an opponent of single-payer "Canadian-style" reforms argued that proposing American adoption of universal public health insurance was tantamount to "selling to the U.S. a product that is about as American as hockey" (Birch 1993, 406). Since 1993 there have been six new National Hockey League (NHL) franchises—all of which are American. In the same period Canada has lost two of its franchises. In 2008 there are now thirty NHL franchises—only six of which are Canadian. In the thirteen seasons before 1993, a Canadian team won the Stanley Cup eight times. Since 1993, there have been fourteen championship NHL hockey franchises—none of which have been Canadian. Viewed from the vantage point of 2008, Birch's 1993 statement emphasizes a crucial point not only about hockey but also about health care.

The Prospects for Convergence in U.S. and Canadian Systems

The development of public health insurance in each country is path dependent—not in the sense that a particular direction of historical development is locked in—but in the sense that no matter which direction public health insurance in either country develops, it will have to start from where it is already. Even if each were to adopt fundamental elements drawn from the other system, each would be building toward that system from a very different starting point. It is true in both cases that, in the vernacular, you can't get there from here.

A stark case in point is the problem of uninsurance evident in the American health care system. Political rhetoric aside, increasing the scope of private health service provision or private funding for health services in Canada will not lead to a system resembling the American mix of categorical public insurance alongside a strong second tier of private, employment-based insurance. Even if Canada were to move closer toward principles enshrined in the American model, there is very little reason to think that moving in this direction, starting from a system of universal coverage, would likely result in the emergence of the uninsurance problem that plagues the U.S. system—although the specter of this eventuality is the most common objection to "Americanizing" reforms in Canadian health care debates.

Conversely, efforts in the United States to strive for universal insurance coverage or even some approximation of a single-payer system are unlikely to lead to health care provision closely resembling the Canadian first-dollar, universal, single-payer model. If the United States is to move toward universal coverage, it will most likely be by expanding existing public programs to a wider range of population and services—leaving much of the current employment-based health insurance system in place. Alternatively, if the United States or, more plausibly, individual American states were to move toward some approximation of a single-payer system, such a system would not likely be based on exclusive public payment for covered services (i.e., excluding coinsurance, user fees, and premiums) nor would the system likely displace physicians practicing completely outside the public system as has largely been the case in the Canadian system.

Health Care Reform in the United States

Health care reform remains an important item on the American political agenda. A decade after the failure of the Clinton proposals, another health care crisis has emerged. This was inevitable largely because none of the incremental reforms in the wake of the Clinton failure have addressed the most pressing problems in the health insurance system—uninsurance, health insurance insecurity, the cost of private health insurance as well as public programs, and the overall costs of the broader health services system (Mayes 2004a, 2004b). In this context, some sort of reform seems inevitable. The question is whether reform will reinforce the existing system or shift health insurance to some new path—possibly one more similar to the Canadian system. The prospects for the latter over the long term may be greater than many observers (and path dependence analysis) might suggest.

It is not credible to argue that institutional fragmentation in the United States dictates particular policy outcomes. The most obvious objection to the argument that the American institutional configuration militates against major government interventions is the enactment of such programs in the New Deal—most notably, Social Security, in which contributory public pensions emerged a full thirty years earlier than it did in Canada. There are notable recent examples. Morone recounts the following exchange: "When Senator Daniel Patrick Moynihan (a twenty-five-year veteran of the welfare wars) greeted David Ellwood (a chairman of President Bill Clinton's welfare task force), the senator cracked, 'So, you've come to do welfare reform. . . . I'll look forward to reading your book about why it failed this time'" (2003, 138). Of course, Moynihan was proven dead wrong. A similar fate may await those who assume that the fragmentation of American political institutions makes any significant health insurance reform impossible.

First, the current constraints on health care reform in the United States might not be as "hard" as they are generally conceived—especially when viewed relative to those of the past. The elements of political culture that now augur against greater government intervention do not appear more rigid or insuperable than they were. This resistance is not of the same magnitude as that generated by the politics of race in the immediate postwar period when government intervention threatened forced integration of health services. Similarly, institutional fragmentation does not pose a significantly greater challenge now than it did when the Medicare program passed. For example, party cohesion is considerably higher than was the case for the Democrats from the 1930s through the late 1960s. A Democratic president in a period of unified government would not likely face the degree of constraint posed by his or her own congressional caucus as faced FDR after about 1938.

Contemporary perceptions of the power of the health insurance, pharmaceutical, and medical services industries mirror perceptions of the power of organized medicine in the late 1940s and 1950s. The present prospects for reform seem less dim if one imagines the image confronting reformers in the late 1950s and early 1960s. The AMA absolutely and vociferously opposed virtually any type of reform. The AMA, the preeminent interest group organization in the United States for over 30 years, had a long history of forestalling public health insurance reform, dating back to 1935. Its power was showcased by its high-powered and visible publicity campaigns, including the 1948 campaign that was the most expensive publicity campaign to that point in history. Yet, by 1965 the administration adopted legislation that represented, in some important senses, a serious defeat for the AMA.

The lesson of this period is not that the AMA was weak but that its power was the result of conjunctures with other powerful causal factors. If the AMA's resistance appeared determinative in the 1930s, it was because the push behind reform was not yet sufficiently powerful and policymakers did not perceive health reform as central to the primary policy problems of the Depression. If its resistance appeared determinative in the late 1940s and 1950s, it was because it was underpinned by a rough balance between forces of reform and those resisting reform—including the powerful resistance of Southern representatives to reforms that could challenge the racial status quo. When this resistance collapsed, so did the apparent power of the AMA. This history suggests the need for caution in attributing power to interest groups (including the interests currently buttressing the existing health insurance system in the United States) and the need for careful analysis of the broader historical context in which this power is exercised.

Second, the history of Medicare and Medicaid in the United States as well as public health insurance programs in Canada compellingly illustrates the degree to which policy can change politics and the malleability of public opinion. Successful expansions of state initiatives for universal health insurance coverage, possibly in tandem with expansions in Medicaid and SCHIP programs, may well shift the center of gravity of public opinion about the appropriate government role in health insurance.

Third, another lesson that emerges from a historical examination of policy reform in the United States concerns the length of time that typically separates the emergence of a policy problem on the political agenda and the adoption of policy. National compulsory health insurance emerged on the agenda thirty years earlier and received presidential support twenty years before significant reform, the Medicare package, was enacted. The most recent round of comprehensive health insurance reform was reignited only sixteen years ago. Major reform within two or three presidential terms after the presidential elections of 2008 would be comparable to the lag that preceded the passage of Medicare. Even in the context of the Canadian parliamentary system, comprehensive reform initially failed. The system that emerged in Canada (which still remains seriously incomplete by the standards of the blueprint for reform in 1945) came about through a halting process that extended public health insurance by service area—losing momentum before coverage was extended to pharmaceuticals, long-term care, and dental care. The development of even this partial public insurance coverage took a long time, with public hospital and medical care insurance coverage being implemented only a quarter of a century later and consolidated more than forty years after the first serious attempt at national-level reform.

Health Care Reform in Canada

The belief that the Canadian system of health care is firmly rooted in some innate, distinctively Canadian set of values does not fit with the historical development of public health insurance in Canada. The degree to which public support of public health insurance has been politically constructed in Canada is marked. The implication is that the lock-in effects created by public opinion have limits as public support can be politically deconstructed or reconstructed. Public support for health care, especially for its role in defining the Canadian social compact as different from the United States, has put serious limits on reform over the twenty years since enhanced free trade with the United States first was seriously debated in Canada. The role that health care has played in this regard, however, was the product of a particular historical conjuncture. Politically linking health care with national unity and national identity must be continually re-created. There is nothing to guarantee that this will continue to be a successful political strategy. Should the public system of health insurance, including effective bans on third-party insurance in various provinces, come to be perceived as an infringement of citizenship rights guaranteed under the Charter, public health insurance may become unmoored from the underpinnings of its public support. Should health insurance, national unity, and national distinctiveness become decoupled, prospects for path-shifting reform will be considerably greater. Proponents of the current system should not take its political underpinnings for granted.

A second lesson from the historical development of Canada's public health insurance is the centrality of the politics of territorial integration. There is little reason to expect that the centrality of territorial politics to the politics of health care in Canada is likely to diminish. Health care continues to touch every single citizen directly in a way that other social programs, such as unemployment insurance, postsecondary education, and even pensions, do not. No program appears likely to displace it in this role. There is little reason to expect (except in the long term) a reversal of the trend in which, within a global knowledge-based economy, the federal government's role has been increasingly constrained while the functions exercised by provincial governments have become increasingly important. Because health care is so central to the relationship between governments and citizens in

Canada and territorial integration is so central to the federal government, the latter will have strong incentives to vigilantly guard its role in this field.

The focus of concern in terms of territorial integration has been Québec, and the direction of development of health services in Québec will continue to play a critical role in the overall trajectory of the Canadian health care system. Thus far, the strategy of provincial diversity within the rubric of an ostensibly unified pan-Canadian system has worked. If, however, Québec goes further in pushing the boundaries of the pan-Canadian system's principles (which it has the constitutional right to do) or if, alternatively, other provinces more vigorously challenge the asymmetrical application of national principles between Québec and the other provinces, there will be tremendous pressure on the system. Territorial politics pose a much greater threat to the disintegration of the pan-Canadian system than does the technical ability of a single-payer system to deliver health services in a timely, equitable, and effective manner that if not for the complications of politics, which cannot be wished away, the latter could almost certainly do.

Conclusion

Of course, there are very tight limits on our ability to peer forward into the future based on the past; nevertheless, doing so with a solid grasp of where we have been is the best that we can do. Despite the difficulties inherent in drawing direct lessons from the cross-border experience with public health insurance, understanding the factors shaping the historical development of public health insurance in the other country is, for observers of health care on both sides of the border, indispensable in understanding the development of public health insurance in their own.

The politics of race played a central role in shaping the development of public health insurance in the United States. Conventional interpretations of America's exceptional development in this regard that rely on political culture, political institutions, or path dependence do not adequately explain the similarities and differences in the historical development in the United States relative to developments in Canada. The example of Canada provides a comparative reference point that highlights the significant role of the politics of race in U.S. developments. It also provides an analogous example of how large-scale processes, such as territorial integration in Canada and the extension of civil rights in the United States, have crucial impacts on policy development. To adequately understand the divergent paths taken by each country in the development of public health insurance, one must factor in the role played by the politics of race in the United States and the politics of territorial integration in Canada.

NOTES

Chapter One

1. For an excellent overview, see Byrd and Clayton (2000, 2002).

2. This view has more recently come under serious challenge (see Béland and Hacker 2004; Béland 2005).

3. The 1980 referendum to pursue "sovereignty-association" had been decisively defeated by 60 percent to 40 percent. In response to the 1995 outcome, the Canadian government enacted legislation outlining the conditions under which a referendum in Québec would provide the Government of Québec with a legal mandate to negotiate secession—legislation that was ruled as constitutional by the Supreme Court of Canada in 1998.

4. As discussed below, the federal government equalizes the fiscal capacity of poorer provinces so that they can provide "reasonably comparable" levels of public service at "reasonably comparable" levels of taxation—a function that, as of 1982, is required by the Canadian Constitution.

5. In regards to Lipset's claims, Marmor aptly notes that "never has so much been claimed with so little evidence" (2002b, 403).

6. Differences in political culture might be reflected in differences in the strength of organized labor in the two countries or in the way that organized labor pursued its interests. Unionization rates were comparable in the two countries across the period in which the crucial differences in public health insurance between the two countries were emerging—being slightly higher in the United States from the mid-1930s into the 1950s and then slightly higher in Canada until they began to diverge markedly in the mid-1970s (see Iton 2000, 7–8, tables 1.1 and 1.2). Differences in unionization rates cannot, by themselves, offer an explanation of differences in the development of public health insurance in the two countries. Furthermore, while there were differences in the orientation of organized labor toward public health insurance in the 1910 and 1920s, in later periods labor adopted the same pro-insurance stance in both countries.

7. Although the president may veto legislation, Congress still retains the power to overturn a presidential veto.

8. Canada's constitution spells out areas of federal jurisdiction, provincial jurisdiction, and concurrent jurisdiction. Any powers not explicitly enumerated in this division of powers are reserved for the federal government—a stark contrast with the American Constitution. The federal government is also given a broad head of power for matters deemed to be related to the maintenance of "peace, order and good government" while the provinces are given a broad head of power for "all matters of a merely local or private nature."

9. To avoid confusion, I use " 'path dependence' " to refer to the ensemble of concepts—critical junctures, sequencing, and positive feedback. The dynamics by which a particular policy direction becomes self-reinforcing, sometimes referred to elsewhere as "path dependence," is referred to here as positive feedback.

10. In Kingdon's conception, these windows of opportunity open when there is a confluence of the distinct problem, policy, and political streams that contribute to policymaking (1984).

11. Orren and Skowronek refer to these collisions or abrasions among distinct realms as "intercurrence" (2004, 113–18; see Pierson 2004, 55–58).

12. Thelen's work is in reference to political institutions; however, these concepts and conceptions of processes of change have been widely adopted in the public policy literature.

13. In an indemnity model of insurance, the individual is insured up to a specified amount to pay for a particular service. This contrasts with a service model in which the service is provided directly by the insurer.

Chapter Two

1. The *Journal of the National Medical Association* and the NAACP's "The Crisis: A Record of the Darker Races" provide a lengthy catalogue of instances of each of the various aspects of racial segregation in health services outlined below.

2. One example was the medical school at Johns Hopkins University, which ostensibly was open to African American students but claimed that no qualified African American students could be found.

3. For example, in Louisiana the blood segregation law made it a misdemeanor for a physician to give a transfusion of blood to a person of a different race without the patient's express permission (Titmuss 1970, 106).

4. Reflecting this, the main report of the CES contained only a very brief reference to health insurance. Instead the CES presented a second report on health insurance directly to the president. The report was never publicly released, received no newspaper coverage, and was ultimately referred for further study (Witte 1963, 189).

5. The bill in Tennessee was the only one to pass (Shearon 1940, 35).

6. In comparison, however, sixty-two bills were proposed with regard to voluntary health insurance (twenty-seven of which passed), and sixty-four bills were proposed with regard to medical assistance for needy persons (twenty-two of which passed).

7. This number refers to bills that proposed health insurance independent of unemployment insurance. Bills in Connecticut (two), Oregon, Missouri, Rhode Island, Washington, and New York (nine) were virtually identical to the model health insurance bill of the American Association for Social Security (the Epstein bill) or based on its earlier 1934 version. While the model bill included both cash benefits as well as medical care coverage, other versions—such as a series of bills in Wisconsin (three) and a bill in New York—provided only for coverage of medical services, with no cash benefits (see Stucke 1952, 1557).

8. The plan "covered employees with incomes below $3,000 per annum (about 90% of the workforce) on a compulsory basis. . . . Payments to doctors would be on a capitation basis to control costs. A tax totaling 3% of payroll, to be shared equally by employers, employees, and the state, would finance the program" (Mitchell 2002, 12).

9. Warren's plan included compulsory coverage of wage earners (earning up to $4,000 per year) and their dependents for both hospital and physician services on a fee-for-service basis paid for by a 3 percent payroll tax shared equally by employers and employees (Mitchell 2002, 19–20).

10. According to Mitchell the failure of the plan was the result of the failure of Warren to "condition" public opinion as well as a failure to prepare the legislature for his plan. (Mitchell 2002, 15). This, according to Mitchell, was crucial as public opinion on health insurance was "fluid": "A 1943 CMA-sponsored poll found that about half the population supported 'socialized' medicine. But it also found that support for a government plan fell sharply if a private alternative were offered" (2002, 15).

11. The Liberal Party platform read as follows: "That is so far as may be practicable, having regard for Canada's financial position, an adequate system of insurance against unemployment, sickness, dependence in old age, and other disability, which would include old age pensions, widow's pensions, and maternity benefit, should be instituted by the Federal Government in conjunction with the Governments of the several provinces; and that on matters pertaining to industrial and social legislation an effort should be made to overcome any question of jurisdiction between the Dominion and the provinces by effective cooperation between the several governments."

12. Ontario was the only province to have undertaken a provincial program of medical relief, which was instituted in 1932. The program subsidized municipal plans that provided partial compensation to physicians providing medical services to the indigent. By 1933 the Ontario Medical Association (OMA) was calling for provincial administration of the program—a request the provincial government would not grant (see Naylor 1986, 65, 82).

13. "Strangely, the report did not see the light of day at all, as the government decided not to release it. Only a typescript of the report, copies of the many briefs submitted, and documents from several American states occupy a file in the provincial archives" (Taylor 1990, 39).

14. For an excellent overview of developments in British Columbia, see Naylor (1986, chapter 4, 58–94).

15. "Contributions by employers were not to exceed 2 percent of their payroll, and those by employees were not to exceed 3 percent of income; the government would contribute on behalf of indigents at one-half the normal rate" (Taylor 1990, 40–41).

16. Letter quoted in Taylor (1990, 41).

Chapter Three

1. Later iterations of the bill (e.g., S. 1320, 1947) were even more expansive, with "coverage extended to encompass groups beyond the purview of social security in 1947, like farmers and the self-employed. Welfare recipients would have their premiums paid by their state welfare agencies" (Poen 1979, 98).

2. The shift from the state-operated system envisioned in earlier proposals (such as the Wagner proposals of 1939) and the federal sponsorship and direction envisioned in the Wagner–Murray–Dingell bill of 1943 have argued to have been the result of a number of factors including Supreme Court decisions on New Deal legislation that appeared to sanction such federal expansion, the support of labor for centralization, and the wartime context that favored centralization (Poen 1979, 32).

3. Providing support for this contention, testimony before a Senate subcommittee in 1949 belied wide discrepancies in the number of hospital beds allocated by race in various states. For example, testimony outlined that, in Mississippi, designated white beds outnumbered designated colored beds by a ratio of two to one—despite the fact that blacks made up 45 percent of the population (U.S. Senate, Committee on Labor and Public Welfare, Subcommittee on Hospital Construction and Local Public Health Units 1949, 116, 164).

4. In August 1949, the day before the NMA convention dealt with the issue of national compulsory health insurance, the AMA appointed the first ever black physician to its House of Delegates. The next day the NMA deferred a motion to support national health insurance (NYT 1949a, 1949g).

5. This position was restated in congressional hearings in 1949 (U.S. Senate, Committee on Labor and Public Welfare, Subcommittee on Health Legislation 1949, 506).

6. Other pieces of legislation proposed at the time that were alleged to be steps to "socialize America" included the Economic Stability Act of 1949, the Brannan plan for subsidizing farm incomes (*Congressional Record* 1950, 2307–9), federal aid to education, and the Truman civil rights program (*Congressional Record* 1951, A4087).

7. As Schiltz notes, "Unfortunately, it is impossible to recover any detailed examination of the public's reasons for opposition to national health insurance" (1970, 135).

8. Of respondents, 47 percent stated that it would be "all right" (Strunk 1946; 1949, 623).

9. While the number of respondents who had heard of the plan increased from 61 percent in January to 71 percent by December 1949, over 60 percent of all respondents still either had not heard of the plan or had no opinion as to the best argument for or against national health insurance.

Chapter Four

1. Lyndon Johnson's full presidential address is available at www.lbjlib.utexas.edu/johnson/archives.hom/speeches.hom/650730.asp. Last visited January 28, 2008.

2. John F. Kennedy, president of the United States, to Dr. W. Montague Cobb, chairman, Council on Medical Education and Hospitals, National Medical Association. Reprinted in the *Journal of the National Medical Association* 54, 4 (July 1962): 501.

3. The effect of the Kerr–Mills Act was limited, and after three years "many states had not acted at all, and five large industrial states, with one third of the nation's population, were receiving 90 percent of the funds" (Starr 1982, 369).

4. As Harris noted, "In an average off-year election, the party in power loses thirty-nine seats in the House and two or three in the Senate. In that year's election, the Democrats lost two seats in the House and picked up four in the Senate. Not a single seat was lost by a candidate who had campaigned for Medicare" (1966, 149). Senator Clinton Anderson, who had cosponsored the medicare bill in 1961, campaigned on the issue of health insurance and won, demonstrating, in his opinion, that "there was widespread support for our notion and that Medicare was not, as the AMA insisted, 'the kiss of political death'" (Anderson 1970, 268; see also S. David 1985, 85).

5. For editorials attributing the delay solely to Mills, see NYT 1964a, NYT 1964b, and NYT 1964c. The first of these editorials charged that "there seems little reason to doubt that a majority of members of both House and Senate are prepared to vote for the Administration's medicare program if they ever get the chance." The final editorial bluntly stated: "The chief reason the country does not now have a medicare program is the one-man blockade exercised for four years by Chairman Wilbur D. Mills of the House Ways and Means Committee."

6. James M. Quigley, assistant secretary, DHEW to Anthony Celebrezze, secretary, DHEW, December 2, 1963. Robert M. Ball Papers, box 114, file 9. Also, Alanson W. Wilcox, general counsel, DHEW to Anthony Celebrezze, secretary, DHEW, June 24, 1963. Robert M. Ball Papers, box 115, folder 1.

7. Quigley to Celebrezze, December 2, 1963.

8. Available online at http://usinfo.state.gov/usa/infousa/laws/majorlaw/civilr19.htm (accessed on April 17, 2007).

9. In conjunction with its strategy of increasing pressure on nonsouthern congressional representatives by portraying them as being allied with the AMA in opposition to the public welfare, the administration had employed a consistent strategy since 1961 of slowly replacing anti-Medicare southern Democrats on the Ways and Means Committee with those who were amenable to the program (Marmor 1970, 54–55). These efforts, by 1964, had brought the

pro-Medicare forces on the committee to within one short of a majority. While important, this strategy was not the key factor in overcoming the reluctance of the committee and Chairman Mills.

10. As such, the exchange is not recorded in the *Congressional Record*. Ball would later recount that this colloquy was the only basis for DHEW's interpretation of congressional intent that Title VI apply to Medicare (NASI 2001, 7).

11. John A. Kenney, National Medical Association, to Robert M. Ball, commissioner of Social Security, December 14, 1962. Robert M. Ball Papers, box 147, file 7.

12. Wilcox to Celebrezze, June 24, 1963.

13. Leaving the administration of Medicaid to the state level is also argued to have enhanced the position of the AMA, which was in a more powerful bargaining position relative to individual states than relative to the federal government (Stevens and Stevens 1974, 354).

14. By 1965 it was estimated that more than half of all nursing home residents received Kerr–Mills payments for nursing home care (Vladeck 1980, 47).

15. Oral comments by Arthur Hess, Restructuring Medicare for the Long Term Project, 2001: 8. Also "Medicare Program: The President's Remarks to Medical and Hospital Leaders Meeting to Prepare for the Launching of the Program, June 15th 1966" from Weekly Compilation of Presidential Documents. Robert M. Ball Papers, box 34, folder 21.

16. In the case of Medicaid, design of payment mechanisms was left to the states. This reopened the issue of compensation for physician services under existing state vendor payment programs. A number of state vendor payments that had previously compensated physicians according to a fixed fee schedule moved to a system based on "usual and customary charges" similar to remuneration under Medicare (Stevens and Stevens 1974, 191).

17. The boycott would have been symbolic as "there was no way for them to carry out this threat . . . for the law provided that if a doctor refused to fill out a Medicare form and, instead, sent his bill to the patient as usual, the patient could collect from the government by simply sending in the doctor's bill and record of its having been paid" (Harris 1966, 217).

18. Certainly, the AMA could have threatened a boycott without risking antitrust prosecution.

19. For additional assessments of federal officials of the role of Medicare in hospital desegregation, see Ball (2001) and Hess (1996).

20. The most likely path for expansion was thought to be initially through the extension of health insurance to children and pregnant mothers (Marmor 2000, 95–96).

21. The Senate Finance report also asserted the programs were having deleterious effects on health insurance provision more generally: "The two programs are also adversely affecting health care costs and financing for the general population" (U.S. Senate, Committee on Finance 1970, 1).

22. Medicaid recipients could not have a cash income greater than 133 percent of AFDC benefits (see Stevens and Stevens 1974, 117–21).

23. A number of federal regulations have slowly been adopted to fill the regulatory void created by the ERISA provision; however, these restrictions remain limited. In 1982 employers who offered health plans to their employees were required to cover certain workers who would otherwise be eligible for Medicare. In 1985 the "Consolidated Omnibus Budget Reconciliation Act [COBRA] required employers to offer, but not subsidize, continuing access to group health plans for workers leaving a job. . . . And in 1996 the Health Insurance Portability and Accountability Act [HIPAA] placed new restrictions on the practices of self-insured plans to encourage portability of benefits across jobs and limit specific exclusions

from coverage. At the same time, Congress added two specific benefit mandates—one requiring minimum levels of coverage for maternity care, the other seeking parity of coverage between mental health services and other medical treatment" (Hacker 2002, 259n155).

24. In part this was because "at the time of its creation, the preemption language applied only to a minority of health plans." However, "corporations and unions quickly responded to the largely unnoticed preemption clause in ERISA, underwriting worker's [*sic*] medical risks on their own to limit cross-subsidization across employee groups and evade state regulations and taxes. By the mid-1980s, roughly half of corporate health plans were self-insured, and the proportion rose to more than two-thirds by the early 1990s" (Hacker 2002, 256–57).

25. As Hacker noted twenty years after the enactment of ERISA, "the few states that have considered more ambitious reforms have found themselves unable to reach many of the privately insured within their borders" (2002, 412). There is, however, considerable controversy over the extent to which ERISA has, in fact, forestalled state reform efforts.

26. See, for example, Murray (1984).

27. Regarding organized labor, see Gottschalk (2000).

Chapter Five

1. As Skocpol explains: "Health care is not a luxury good that people do without. When people finally show up in emergency rooms, costs simply escalate and get shifted around" (1996, 17).

2. For an overview of critical design decisions, see Skocpol (1996, 65–72).

3. The Medicare-related proposals included the extension of coverage for prescriptions drugs and long-term care.

4. The quotes from Clinton are taken from Skocpol (1996, 45, 112).

5. This particular survey question was chosen because it could be expected to be sensitive to changes in attitudes to policy related to race without being explicitly based on racial attitudes, which might elicit a high level of respondent reluctance to be forthright.

6. In keeping with these findings, 58 percent of respondents in 1994 agreed that "until racial minorities shape up and realize they can't get a free ride, there will be little improvement in race relations in America" (National Conference of Christians and Jews 1994). In 1995, 93 percent of respondents agreed that "low-income minorities need to take more individual responsibility and become less dependent on government" (Harvard University and Kaiser Family Foundation 1995).

7. A decade and a half after its introduction, there are over a dozen standard works on the Clinton health reforms—not one of which considers the role played by the politics of race in shaping health care reform in this period. In her review of the existing literature explaining the failure of the Clinton reforms, Quadagno notes, "Others blamed more enduring features of American politics—the institutional structure of the state, antistatist values, or racist sentiments" (2005, 200). However, of the seven references cited for this trio of explanations, only one refers to the politics of race—Morone's "Nativism, Hollow Corporations and Managed Competition."

8. While Iton presents data on the differences in uninsured status by race, he does not provide any evidence relating to popular perceptions of the uninsured, public perceptions regarding the scope of the problem of uninsurance, or analysis of media coverage of the issue.

9. In contrast with the mass of evidence presented by Gilens in regard to welfare reform, Iton does not offer any evidence of the conflation of health insurance programs and welfare by the media, policymakers, or other political actors.

10. Schlesinger and Lee's analysis controls for "other ongoing changes in economic well-being and social characteristics" (1994, 315).

11. While African Americans were 10 percent more likely than whites to support a governmental role in health policy (a statistically significant difference), they were much more supportive of programs for the poor (18.4 percent higher than whites) and government involvement in domestic policy in general (20.3 percent higher than whites) (Schlesinger and Lee 1994, 310). These regressions hold age, sex, education, marital status, income, employment status, and rural vs. urban residency constant. This pattern of difference remained stable across the period under consideration—1975 to 1989.

12. A similar poll question in 1999 reinforces the conclusion that Americans tend to overestimate the degree of uninsurance: 32 percent of respondents estimated the rate of uninsurance at below 20 percent (with 24 percent estimating it correctly between 11 percent and 20 percent), and 56 percent of respondents estimated the uninsurance rate at more than 25 percent of the American population (Families USA and Health Insurance Association of America 1999, Question 22).

13. Prior to 1993 there are no survey questions that specifically ask about the ability of the "uninsured" to get needed medical care; rather, the questions focus on the ability of the "poor" to get such care. Starting in 1993, polls began asking respondents about their perceptions of the access of the uninsured to needed medical care. In 1993, while 41 percent of respondents believed that the uninsured could not get needed medical care, a slightly higher proportion of respondents (43 percent) believed that the uninsured were still able to get care (Robert Wood Johnson Foundation and Harvard School of Public Health 1993). The fact that a higher proportion of respondents in 1993 believed that the uninsured could receive needed medical services than the proportion believing that the poor could receive needed medical services is indicative of the belief that some proportion of the uninsured is made up of the nonpoor who are voluntarily uninsured.

14. Support for "protecting against coverage loss" as a goal of national health reform at 83 percent marked a statistically significant difference with the other three goals—universal coverage, containing costs, and ensuring quality.

15. Reviewing public opinion polling in regard to health and welfare programs from 1975 to 1989, Schlesinger and Lee note: "Although the late 1980s saw increased attention to disparities in access and health outcomes between white and various minority groups, little is known about the extent to which various government health programs are racially identified. . . . Virtually nothing is known about racial identification of health programs by the general public" (1994, 329).

16. William J. Clinton (1994, State of the Union Address).

17. Nor was a link between health reform and welfare drawn in the media except in the limited coverage of the last-ditch efforts by proponents of reform to argue, in the proposal's dying days, that health care reform was necessary for successful welfare reform.

18. Iton argues that "assumptions rooted in racial understandings have been internalized and incorporated into the process associated with making health care policy and public policy in general. The president who came in pledging to 'end welfare as we know it,' given the class and racial connotations associated with that promise, was not likely to have a strong mandate (or the confidence) to undertake comprehensive health care reform or to make health coverage for the uninsured a national priority" (2000, 169). While the analysis above provides a significantly different perspective on the link between race and health care reform than that offered by Iton, it agrees with his conclusion that "Clinton's racial calculations . . . meant that he would have very little leeway with which to fashion a feasible and effective health care package" (2000, 170).

Chapter Six

1. The federal government managed to avoid having to implement conscription until late 1944.

2. Similar to the fate of certain elements of the Roosevelt New Deal, the Employment and Social Insurance Act had been struck down by the Supreme Court of Canada—its constitutionality having been challenged by the Province of Ontario (Taylor 1990, 44). In response, the federal government set up the Royal Commission on Dominion–Provincial Relations (Rowell–Sirois) in 1937, which issued its report in 1940.

3. The report would note: "We emphasize . . . the importance of limiting the transfer of jurisdiction to the Dominion that what is strictly necessary" (Royal Commission on Dominion–Provincial Relations 1939, 13).

4. According to the commission report, "Health insurance differs profoundly from unemployment insurance and contributory old age pensions. . . . Unlike unemployment insurance, health insurance is not subject to wide variations in demand; the risks are more easily estimated, and more constant. It is not subject to cyclical fluctuations, or sudden emergencies making widespread and prolonged drains on reserve funds. . . . Unlike contributory old age pensions, health insurance is not a compulsory saving scheme requiring individual accounts over many working years. . . . No serious problems of reserves or of bookkeeping for a migratory labour force are thus likely to arise. We see, therefore, no insuperable obstacle to the establishment of health insurance by a province" (Royal Commission on Dominion–Provincial Relations 1939, 42).

5. As an influential study commissioned by the Royal Commission would note, "no federal government will ever have the courage to sanction the withdrawal of a grant from any one of the provinces. The good-will of each province is very important to the Dominion administration when there are only nine. . . . A government at Ottawa will not withdraw a grant from a government supported by its party in one of the provinces, because it cannot risk internal dissension. It will scarcely dare to withdraw a grant from a government of a different political faith because of the capital that could be made of its actions by the opposition. . . . Therefore the power to withhold a grant is virtually only a paper power. . . . It could not be used safely in Canada . . ." (Corry 1939, 35).

6. The Heagerty report was released simultaneously with the Marsh report (Report on Social Security for Canada), which dealt with social security more broadly but also recommended "a comprehensive system of health insurance, including all medical, dental, pharmaceutical, and optometrist's services, provincially administered but jointly financed by the federal and provincial governments with contributions from the insured population" (Guest 1997, 112).

7. The Heagerty report proposed universal coverage for a comprehensive range of health benefits including medical, dental, pharmaceutical, hospital, and nursing services. However, it proposed allowing provinces to limit compulsory insurance to individuals under a certain income threshold. Programs would be financed through a mix of premiums and federal and provincial contributions with the provinces paying premiums of the indigent. There was also to be a dedicated health insurance tax of 3 to 5 percent based on marital status. See Guest (1997, 131).

8. A Gallup poll taken in March 1944 reported an 80 percent affirmative response to the question "Would you contribute to a national hospital–medical insurance plan?" (Taylor 1990, 54).

9. Another unresolved issue was tax rental—an arrangement by which the provinces during wartime had ceded certain areas of provincial taxation to the federal government

in return for unconditional federal grants. The agreement proposed an extension of these arrangements. Both Ontario and Québec opposed the proposals. The former disagreed with the structure and level of proposed federal compensation for ceded tax room (Naylor 1986, 133–4). However, the premier of Québec, Maurice Duplessis, objected on the basis of constitutional principle—arguing that the proposals undermined the federal–provincial division of powers enshrined in the British North America Act, Canada's central constitutional document at the time.

10. Premier Maurice Duplessis quoted in Taylor (1987, 62–63).

11. In this regard, the federal government's abandonment of a more unified approach to provincial plans before convening the Dominion–Provincial conference was a "serious disappointment" for the CMA (Taylor 1987, 46). This is in striking contrast to the case in the United States, where the medical profession was strongly predisposed toward control by state governments.

12. The CMA shift was followed by similar reversals by both the CHA and CLIA (Taylor 1990, 84).

13. The range of options was similarly impressive, with physician and hospital plans tending to offer service plans (i.e., direct provision of an agreed-upon set of services) while private insurers tended to offer indemnity plans (i.e., providing a set fee for a given medical procedure with copayments and deductibles). Private insurers offered both group plans as well as individual plans and, unlike prepayment plans of medical and hospital associations, were typically experience-rated and could often offer considerably lower premiums than Blue Cross or Blue Shield.

14. All four parties in the 1949 federal election were committed to health insurance (although they varied widely in terms of specifics). However, health insurance was given minor emphasis by the two major parties (Taylor 1990, 83–84).

15. In addition to Saskatchewan and British Columbia, Alberta also developed a plan of provincial government subsidies for municipal tax-financed hospital insurance schemes rather than a province-wide compulsory hospital insurance plan as was the case in Saskatchewan and British Columbia. Under the Alberta Municipal Hospital Plan (1950) individual municipalities could offer tax-financed hospital care to municipal rate payers and nonrate payers who elected to pay premiums (Taylor 1990, 78). Newfoundland, which entered Canada in 1950, had its own system of public health care that was unique. In the outports of Newfoundland (with a population just under half of the total provincial population), the provincial government provided hospital and medical services through provincially owned hospitals and salaried physicians through a plan that required a modest annual premium (Taylor 1990, 80).

16. According to C. Rufus Rorem, a researcher for the U.S. Committee on the Costs of Medical Care (CCMC) who studied the Saskatchewan municipal doctor system in the period, "Each of the municipalities which has adopted the municipal doctor system had already had unsatisfactory experiences with the conventional methods of private practice. . . . In several instances a local physician placed before the municipality the alternative of employing him on an annual salary or having him move to another community." The CCMC in the United States recommended that a similar program be implemented in particular areas in the United States.

17. An important innovation in 1941 was a municipal system of tax prepaid hospital and physician care that allowed residents to choose from any doctor or hospital anywhere in the province (as opposed to limiting choice to salaried doctors in that particular municipality) (Houston 2002, 78).

18. Full results of the survey are reported in the *Saskatchewan Medical Quarterly*.

19. The CCF philosophy, although it clearly could be considered a democratic socialist party, was at root an extension of the "social gospel" vision. This vision originated in the United States; it was influential after the Civil War and peaked during the Progressive Era (from the turn of the century to the end of World War II). For an overview of the social gospel doctrine in the United States, see Morone (2004).

20. Under the heading "Socialized Health Services—Publicly Organized Health, Hospital and Medical Services," the Regina Manifesto states: "Health services should be made at least as freely available as are educational services today. But under a system which is still mainly one of private enterprise the costs of proper medical care, such as the wealthier members of society can easily afford, are at present prohibitive for great masses of the people. A properly [i.e., publicly] organized system of public health services including medical and dental care . . . should be extended to all our people in both rural and urban areas" (CCF 1933).

21. Thus, for example, the decision to make the plan a contributory social insurance program based on premiums was in direct response to the Green Book proposals, which emphasized premiums (Taylor 1990, 70).

22. The provincial legislation was passed in February 1946, and the federal–provincial negotiations ended in failure in early May 1946 (Taylor 1990, 58).

23. At the outset of these reforms, the Liberals held thirty-four of forty-seven seats (with the CCF holding seven) having received 42 percent of the popular vote in comparison with 32 percent for the CCF. In the 1937 election, in which the health reforms were a central issue, the Liberals again bested the CCF by a comfortable margin (37 percent compared to 29 percent), and the CCF did not pick up any seats although the Liberals lost eight to the Conservative Party.

24. After the 1941 election, the Liberals and Conservatives ran a coalition government with the CCF in opposition. The 1941 election outcomes were as follows: Liberals, 33 percent of the popular vote and twenty-one of forty-eight seat; CCF, 33 percent of the popular vote and fourteen seats; Conservatives, 31 percent of the vote and twelve seats (British Columbia 2005). Subsequently, in the 1945 and 1949 elections, the Liberals and Conservatives ran in the election as a coalition party. The 1945 election outcomes were as follows: Coalition, 56 percent of the popular vote and thirty-seven of forty-eight seats; CCF, 38 percent of the popular vote and ten seats. The 1949 election outcomes were as follows: Coalition, 61 percent of the popular vote and thirty-nine of forty-eight seats; CCF, 35 percent of the popular vote and seven seats (British Columbia 2005).

25. A weak form of equalization was implicit in the 1952 federal–provincial agreements. Explicit equalization in its contemporary form was first included in the 1957–62 tax revenue agreements.

Chapter Seven

1. Newspaper headlines reported "Provinces Win" (Taylor 1987, 127).

2. The governing federal Liberals had invoked closure and forced passage of legislation approving the construction of a trans-Canada pipeline by interests closely connected with the governing Liberal Party despite strong parliamentary and public opposition.

3. The actual matching formula was based on a blend of "25 percent of the national per capita cost plus 25 percent of the provincial per capita cost" (Taylor 1990, 94). "Every essential requirement for the operation of a program was prescribed by the federal government. The provincial government must establish a hospital planning division; it must license, inspect, and supervise hospitals and maintain adequate standards; it must approve hospitals'

budgets; it must approve the purchase of equipment by hospitals; it must collect the prescribed statistics and submit the required reports, and the province must make insurance service available to all residents on uniform terms and conditions" (Taylor 1990, 93). This last condition "effectively prevented any province from adopting the CMA–CLIA proposal of subsidizing individuals to enable them to pay premiums to the voluntary plans or commercial insurance" (Taylor 1990, 94).

4. The HIDS legislation did not receive CMA endorsement and, furthermore, was subjected to open opposition from the insurance industry as well as the Canadian Association of Chambers of Commerce, among others (Taylor 1990, 92).

5. The provinces, of course, argued that coinsurance payments should be considered a provincial contribution and thus be eligible for federal matching (Taylor 1987, 153).

6. The federal position was only that provincial hospital plans should limit coinsurance fees so that they did not place an "excessive" financial burden on patients (Taylor 1987, 135).

7. Thus, Taylor adjusts the data to include only those provinces without a public health insurance program. As a result hospital benefit coverage in Canada in 1952 increases from 37.6 percent to 43.7 percent (Taylor 1987, 65).

8. While Frost was philosophically predisposed toward private market options, he was particularly inimical to health insurance carriers after two of his own personal health insurance policies were canceled. See Taylor (1987, esp. 154).

9. The following draws from Taylor (1987, 110–24).

10. The largest fifteen firms accounted for over 75 percent of gross premium income for medical insurance in Canada in 1961 and only 38 percent in the United States in 1958 (Tuohy 1999, 50).

11. At the first opportunity following Douglas's speech, the College of Physicians and Surgeons unanimously passed a resolution avowing that "medical care has always been readily available to the public regardless of ability to pay, and that no one has ever been denied medical attention because of his financial position"; "we firmly believe that the standards of medical services to the people will deteriorate under such a system"; and "we oppose the introduction of a compulsory government-controlled, province-wide medical care plan and declare our support of, and the extension of health and sickness benefits through indemnity and service plans" (Taylor 1990, 100–101).

12. As a result of this compromise, doctors had a number of choices of ways to practice: (a) receiving direct payments from the commission as payment in full (either salary or fee for service); (b) billing through a voluntary agency (and accepting billing as payment in full); (c) billing payments at doctors' sole discretion (providing an itemized list so that the patient could apply to the commission for reimbursement from the minimum fee schedule); (d) practice entirely for private fees (no itemized statement required) (Taylor 1990, 125–26). Initially it appeared as if the voluntary agencies (option B) would become a key component of the new system. Direct billing of the government, however, came to supercede billing through voluntary agencies: "In 1963, the proportion of physicians billing the commission directly was minimal, amounting to only 21.5 percent. By 1970 this proportion had increased to 51.5 percent, with the proportion billed through the prepayment plans declining from 68.0 percent to 40.5. With the proportion continuing to decline, in 1988 all physicians' claims were sent directly to the commission" (Taylor 1990, 129).

Chapter Eight

1. The territorial challenges facing the federal state were not limited to those emanating from Québec. As contemporary observers noted at the time, even had Québec remained

quiescent, "the pressures for decentralization have been so fired up by resurgent provincialism that many have questioned the very survival of the federal government as a decisive body" (Black and Cairns 1966, 34).

2. Hacker argues that while pressure for a national program came from the demands of the provinces, the "strongest pressures for action came from the exigencies of the Liberal Party's minority status in parliament" (Hacker 1998, 103, 104).

3. Regarding the former interpretation, see Newman (1968, 412) and La Marsh (1969, 86). Regarding the latter, see Hacker (1998, 103) and Maioni (1998, 162).

4. For Tuohy the shifting of the locus of reform efforts from the federal level to the provincial level in Canada (following the failure of federal health insurance reforms in 1945) appears to have been sufficiently natural that it requires no explanation. For her, what requires explanation is why a similar shift did not take place in the United States—an outcome she attributes to strategic calculation on the part of reformers.

5. The Ontario bill was introduced in 1963 but, instead of being passed, was referred to an independent commission. After extensive public hearings, the commission recommended amendments that included coverage for the indigent (in addition to providing subsidies for low-income earners.) The plan was finally passed in 1966 as the Ontario Medical Services Insurance Plan (OMSIP). A similar plan had also been adopted in British Columbia with the creation of the British Columbia Medical Plan (BCMP) in 1965.

6. Tom Kent, principal assistant to Prime Minister Lester B. Pearson, interview with author, April 2005.

7. Ibid.

8. The CMA executive met with the minister of health and prime minister in June 1965 (Taylor 1990, 141).

9. When asked about the apparent support in public opinion polling for a voluntary plan rather than a compulsory plan, Tom Kent emphasized that senior policymakers did not put much stock in public opinion polls—believing that the answers were largely shaped by the way the questions were asked. They believed that, in the last analysis, a straight public plan was "what people would vote for." As Kent points out, the real evidence of public support for the proposal was that it was voted for unanimously in the House of Commons. Kent, interview.

10. Ibid.

11. For an overview of these principles, see chapter 9. The federal contribution would match total spending by all provinces with this total amount being divided among provinces on a per capita basis.

12. Rather than calling for federal financial aid for health care (or any other specific program area), the Québec government called for the federal government to "make it easier for provinces to exercise their constitutional powers, for example, by rectifying the present system of sharing revenue sources in Canada" (Lésage quoted in Taylor 1990, 147). This continues to be the position of the Québec government in 2008.

13. The importance of symbolic politics is compellingly argued and illustrated in Edelman's classic work, *The Symbolic Uses of Politics*.

14. Kent, interview.

15. Vertical fiscal imbalance refers to the situation by which provincial jurisdictional responsibilities are significantly greater than provincial powers of taxation.

16. In Kent's view this would require asymmetry with regard to Québec. Kent, interview.

17. In addition, the benefits would be taxable in order to make the overall system more progressive. Kent, interview.

18. Ibid.

19. At the same time, Kennedy administration policy advisers also were discussing the idea of Kiddie Care, which was seen to be the natural complement of Medicare—a development of which Canadian policymakers such as Kent were well aware. Ibid.

20. The Hall Commission was appointed in mid-1961 and issued its report three years later, in mid-1964.

21. The report recommended public insurance coverage of a comprehensive range of services including medical services; dental services for children, expectant mothers, and public assistance recipients; prescription drug services; optical services for children and public assistance recipients; prosthetic services; and home care services.

22. Kent, interview.

23. Ibid.

24. Ibid.

25. Ibid. At the time Canada was debating the adoption of a new flag to replace the existing Dominion flag, which incorporated the Union Jack.

26. According to Kent, far more than people appreciated, there was a real alliance between the Lésage and Pearson governments (Kent, interview). According to Peter C. Newman, "Pearson's main policy preoccupation was his attempt to sponsor some kind of accommodation between Québec and the rest of the country" (Newman 1968, 45).

27. Québec Premier Bertrand was resigned: "Ottawa has placed us in a position where we might be one of the last provinces to sign. . . . Either Quebec joins the programme, and thus flies squarely in the face of the Canadian constitution, or else we do not join up and thus deprive our people of a lot of money to which they have the right. What does one do in a case like this? Don't we have to be realistic and make the best of the situation, that is, sign the agreement with Ottawa, counting on its being the last time?" (Taylor 1987, 392).

28. Initially the specialists defied the legislative order but ultimately went back to work "under protest" because of the political crisis precipitated by the FLQ (Taylor 1987, 408–10). In the event, the government did not remove the opting-out clause but did remove the provision allowing for financial compensation (Taylor 1987, 402).

29. The crisis was precipitated in October 1970 when the radical *independentiste* FLQ kidnapped British Trade Commissioner James Cross and kidnapped and murdered Québec's labor minister, Pierre Laporte.

30. As the value of tax points varies from province to province depending on the strength of the provincial tax base, these tax points would be equalized to the national average. Second, the cash component included an escalator tied to per capita GNP.

31. As Taylor notes, "The media had been focusing on the issue, of course, since mid-1978. So heated became the issue that, three public inquiries were launched, the first in 1979" (Taylor 1990, 158).

32. In Alberta 43 percent of all doctors were estimated to be extra-billing as of 1983.

33. Ed Broadbent, 1998. http://www.sfu.ca/mediapr/sfnews/1998/Jan22/quebec.html.

34. In addition, the federal minister of national health and welfare "pointed to the interregional transfers implicit in federal social programs that would disappear." (Banting 1995, 287).

35. Patriation refers to the process of shifting the venue for amending the Canadian constitution from the British Parliament in Westminster to Canada.

36. Another notable nation-building initiative was the National Energy Program of 1980.

37. Extra-billing, often referred to as balance-billing in the United States, occurs when a physician receives a fee for a service from the public insurance program but also bills the patient directly for an amount over and above the fee paid by the public program. While the

act allowed the province to collect premiums for the public plan, access to services could not be restricted on the basis of unpaid premiums (Guest 1997, 212).

38. Most notably was the Québec practice of covering health services received by Québec residents in another province only if covered by (and to the amount covered by) the Québec plan, which clearly violates the principle of portability.

Chapter Nine

1. In a 2000 poll, just under 60 percent of respondents felt that the federal government "should ensure that all Canadians, no matter where they live, have access to similar levels of health care services (Mendelsohn 2001, 77).

2. Taken from the Public Citizen webpage at http://www.citizen.org/trade/nafta/ (accessed on April 20, 2005).

3. The argument has been that the investor protection provisions of NAFTA ensure that, if provincial governments open up certain services to private provision (whether privately or publicly funded), they will have to allow American firms to provide these services. If those provincial governments subsequently wish to return to public provision of those services, they would have to compensate these American firms for appropriated profits.

4. The federal changes placed a cap on total federal contributions. As the value of tax points rise with growth in the economy, tax points would, over time, comprise a larger and larger proportion of overall transfers and cash transfers, which would make up the difference between the value of the tax points and the capped total, would shrink—eventually reaching zero. This issue was resolved by the federal implementation of a floor on the cash component of the CHST transfers, which was an attempt to draw a balance between minimizing fiscal contributions and maintaining a federal ability to claim credit for the politically popular aspects of Canadian medicare.

5. The federal government penalized British Columbia in early 1994 for allowing extra-billing by physicians. In late 1995, the federal government began levying penalties against Alberta for allowing private clinics to charge facility fees with the province retracting the policy six months later. For a good overview, see Boase (2001).

6. Struck in 1994 by the newly elected Liberal government and reporting in 1997, the National Forum on Health (NFH) recommended maintaining the key features of the Canadian health care system. These recommendations included maintaining full public funding for medically necessary services, maintaining the single-payer model, and supporting the five principles of the Canada Health Act while moving away from the fee-for-service mode of remuneration. (In regard to the latter, see National Forum on Health, 1997b, 23.) These various goals would require, according to the NFH, "a significant and ongoing financial contribution through federal transfers" that "must be stable and predictable over time" (National Forum on Health 1997b, 21). Furthermore, the NFH recommended extending universal public insurance coverage to home care (including post-acute, chronic, and palliative care) and universal first-dollar coverage for pharmaceuticals (National Forum on Health 1997b, 11–12).

7. While the accord committed governments to many of the same principles as outlined in the Health Accord (2000), in many cases, the specific commitments were more clearly laid out. These included provision in regards to common performance indicators as well as setting specific targets, such as a commitment to access (24/7).

8. The Conservative Party of Canada was formed in late 2003 as a result of the merger of the Progressive Conservative Party of Canada (which itself had roots back to Confederation in 1867) and the Canadian Alliance (formerly the Reform Party, which had been formed

as a Western regional splinter group of the Progressive Conservatives in 1987). As of 2004, the Conservative Party held 78 of 301 seats in the House of Commons and, as the largest opposition party in the House of Commons, formed the Official Opposition.

9. The following information on specific commitments is drawn from Office of the Prime Minister (2004a).

10. The provincial premiers, somewhat disingenuously, called on the federal government to assume "full responsibility" for a "truly national plan" of comprehensive coverage for prescription drugs (Council of the Federation 2004). The federal preference was clearly for a shared-cost system by which the federal government could claim a central role without shouldering the full burden of cost or administration.

11. This term refers to the increasingly frequent practice of having agreements signed by the nine provinces and federal government with an asterisk beside the title indicating that, although the Government of Québec agrees with the objectives of the program, the agreement does not apply to the Province of Québec.

12. While the health care summit was taking place, the first-ever completely private emergency clinic in Québec announced that it would be opening the following month.

13. In the 2004 federal election, the Conservative Party's leader, Stephen Harper, candidly admitted on national television that his advisers had cautioned him not to talk even about the prospects of private provision of publicly funded health services—in stark contrast to the electoral strategies of the Reform Party in 1997 and Canadian Alliance in 2000. Rather than simply avoiding the subject, the Conservative Party of Canada by 2006 adopted the tactic of strongly championing the principles of the CHA.

Chapter Ten

1. Legislation and program details are available online at http://www.lawlib.state.ma.us/healthinsurance.html (accessed on April 16, 2007).

2. Expenditures on hospitals and physicians compose 29.9 percent and 12.9 percent of total health spending, respectively. Remaining expenditures comprise drugs (16.7 percent), other professionals (14.6 percent), other institutions (9.6 percent), and miscellaneous other expenditures (19.8 percent). From CIHI website, http://secure.cihi.ca/cihiweb/dispPage.jsp?cw_page = statistics_results_topic_macrospend_e&cw_topic = Health percent20Spending&cw_subtopic = Macropercent20Spending (accessed on March 30, 2005).

3. Insurance coverage by population for 2003 was as follows: employer-provided (54 percent), Medicaid (13 percent), Medicare (12 percent), individual (5 percent), and uninsured (16 percent). From Kaiser Family Foundation Statehealthfacts.org, http://www.state healthfacts.kff.org / cgi-bin / healthfacts.cgi?action = compare&category = Health + Coverage + percent26 + Uninsured&subcategory = Insurance + Status&topic = Distribution + by + In surance + Status (accessed on March 30, 2005).

4. For example, "states are now required to set reimbursement rates high enough so that Medicaid services will actually be available to recipients, at least to the extent that they are available to other residents in the state. Health care providers cannot charge Medicaid patients additional fees above these amounts" (Rom 1999, 353).

5. Despite their significance, these expenditures are not generally included in calculations of public health expenditures and are not included in the comparisons of public health expenditures presented in this chapter.

6. As a result of ERISA provisions, states since 1974 have not possessed the legislative authority to enact universal single-payer health care: "current federal law preempts their authority to reform the self-insured portion of the market, which accounts for about half of

all insured workers. A single-payer system would have to be national, or at least it would require the lifting of federal constraints from the states" (Fox and Inglehart 1995).

7. This last condition also applied to individual insurance plans.

8. Despite this, the role of state governments has been downplayed in health care reform debates in the United States: "Rarely heard in the debate over health care reform is a discussion of health care politics at the state level. This lack of analysis is surprising. Not only do state treasuries fund a large share of the nation's health care bills, but also state officials play a key policy role" (Sparer 1994, 430).

9. This discussion relies on the insurance status of children under eighteen in order to avoid distortions caused by "voluntary" uninsured status, which is more common among young, single adults.

10. In Canada the arbitrary level of population coverage initially required for a program to be deemed "universal" was 90 percent. By these standards, twenty-two states have achieved universal health insurance coverage for children under eighteen.

11. Such differences may be explained in part by factors such as the increased costs of serving a province with a sparse population distribution.

12. Canadian Institute for Health Information (CIHI), see http://secure.cihi.ca/cihiweb/splash.html.

13. For a good overview, see Canadian Institute for Health Information, 2004, Appendix: Comparison of Provincial and Territorial Drug Subsidy Programs.

14. Based on data drawn from Canadian Institute for Health Information, 2004, Series B: Expenditure on Drugs by Type, by Source of Finance, and as a Share of Public, Private, and Total Health Expenditure, by Province/Territory, 1985–2004, pages 61–113.

15. As Raffel, Raffel, and Raffel note: "Though uninsured, most of the 38–40 million are able to get needed medical care through hospital emergency departments, which, by law, are not permitted to deny care" (1997, 278).

16. "Indemnity" plans provide reimbursement for costs incurred in obtaining a given range of covered medical services. "Service" plans directly provide a range of specified medical services.

17. The following section is not intended as an overview of existing surveys of perceptions of quality in the two countries. Rather, it relies almost exclusively on the seven-part (as of April 2005) series of surveys designed by researchers at the Harvard School of Public Health and Commonwealth Fund, undertaken by Harris Interactive, and published annually in *Health Affairs* (Blendon et al., 2001, 2002, 2003).

18. The following discussion draws on Blendon et al. (2002).

19. Blendon et al. (2002) do not provide a breakdown of perceptions of excellent/very good care by both income and insurance status although they do provide such a breakdown for perceptions of fair/poor quality care.

20. A major initiative in this regard has been undertaken by the Commonwealth Fund aimed at producing cross-national comparative indicators of health system quality based on objective outcome measures. The following discussion is drawn from Commonwealth Fund (2004).

21. The Commonwealth Fund's International Working Group on Quality Indicators also includes suicide rates and smoking rates in their consideration of avoidable events. I do not include them here as avoidance of these events is only tangentially related to the health care system as traditionally defined.

22. The Commonwealth Fund's International Working Group on Quality Indicators also includes asthma mortality rates (for persons aged five through thirty-nine) although no data

on this indicator are available for Canada as well as the acute myocardial infarction (heart attack) survival rate for which there are no data for the United States.

23. The United States has just under two-thirds of the number of mamographs per capita (OECD 2006).

24. The Commonwealth Fund's International Working Group (CFIWG) on Quality Indicators classifies "sicker adults" as respondents who "reported being in fair or poor health, having had a serious illness, being hospitalized or having had major surgery in the past two years" (Commonwealth Fund 2004).

25. The following discussion draws on Blendon et al. (2003). Unfortunately, the Blendon et al. report, which examines the responses of sicker adults, does not break U.S. respondents down by insurance status, and as a result, these data must be interpreted with caution. However, the size of the uninsured respondent pool is sufficiently small as to have only limited impacts on U.S. totals.

26. These estimates exclude insurance industry personnel.

REFERENCES

AHA. *See* American Hospital Association.

Albright, Robert C. 1949. 81st led to water, made to drink. *Washington Post*, October 16, B1.

American Hospital Association. 2005. *Hospital statistics 2005*. Chicago: Health Forum.

Anderson, Clinton P. 1970. *Outsider in the Senate: Senator Anderson's memoirs*. New York: World Publishing.

Anderson, Odin W. 1951. Compulsory medical care insurance, 1910–1950. In *Annals of the American Academy of Political and Social Science: Medical care for Americans,* ed. Franz Goldmann and Hugh R. Leavell, 106–13. Philadelphia: American Academy of Political and Social Science.

Arkansas Democrat. 1964. Social reform forced on the sick. March 14.

Armstrong, Pat, and Hugh Armstrong with Claudia Fegan. 1998. *Universal health care: What the United States can learn from the Canadian experience.* New York: New York Press.

Atkinson, Graham, W. David Helms, and Jack Needleman. 1997. State trends in hospital uncompensated care. *Health Affairs* (July/August): 233.

Ball, Robert M. 1995. What Medicare's architects had in mind. *Health Affairs*, 14 (Winter): 62–72.

———. 2001. Interview with Robert Ball, former Social Security Commission, 1962–73. *Social Security Administration Oral History Collections.* November. Available at www.ssa .gov/history/orals/balloralhistory.html.

Banting, Keith G. 1987. *The welfare state and Canadian federalism,* 2nd ed. Kingston and Montréal: McGill-Queen's University Press.

———. 1995. The welfare state as statecraft: Territorial politics and Canadian social policy. In *European social policy: Between fragmentation and integration,* eds. Stephan Leibfried and Paul Pierson. Washington, DC: Brookings Institution.

Banting, Keith G., and Stan Corbett. 2002. Health policy and federalism: An introduction. In *Health Policy and Federalism: A Comparative Perspective on Multi-Level Governance,* ed. Keith G. Banting and Stan Corbett, 1–38. Montréal and Kingston: McGill-Queen's University Press.

Barer, Morris L., and Robert G. Evans. 1992. Interpreting Canada: Models, mind-sets, and myths. *Health Affairs* (Spring 1992).

Beardsley, Edward H. 1987. *A history of neglect: Health care for blacks and mill workers in the twentieth-century South.* Knoxville: University of Tennessee Press.

Beauchamp, Dan E. 1996. *Health Care reform and the battle for the body politic.* Philadelphia: Temple University Press.

Béland, Daniel. 2005. *Social Security: History and politics from the New Deal to the privatization debate.* Lawrence: University of Kansas Press.

Béland, Daniel, and Jacob S. Hacker. 2004. Ideas, private institutions and American welfare state 'exceptionalism': The case of health and old-age insurance, 1915–1965. *International Journal of Social Welfare* 13 (2004): 42–54.

Berkowitz, Edward D. 1995. *Mr. Social Security: The life of Wilbur J. Cohen.* Lawrence: University of Kansas Press.

———. 2003. *Robert Ball and the politics of Social Security.* Madison: University of Wisconsin Press.

Birch, Stephen. 1993. Canadian social welfare system goals seen in an American frame of reference. *Canadian Journal on Aging* 12, 3 (1993): 402–6.

Black, Edwin R., and Alan C. Cairns. 1966. A different perspective on Canadian federalism. *Canadian Public Administration* 9, 1 (March): 31–49.

Blendon, Robert J., and K. Donelan. 1990. Special report: The public and the emerging debate over national health insurance. *New England Journal of Medicine* 323, 3 (July): 208–212.

Blendon, Robert J., Cathy Schoen, Karen Donelan, Robin Osborn et al. 2001. Physicians' views on quality of care: A five-country comparison. *Health Affairs* 20, 3 (May/June): 233–44.

Blendon, Robert J., Cathy Schoen, Catherine M. DesRoches, Robin Osborn, Kimberly L. Scoles, and Kinga Zapert. 2002. Inequities in health care: A five-country study. *Health Affairs* 21, 3 (May/June): 182–204.

Blendon, Robert J., Cathy Schoen, Catherine DesRoches, Robin Osborn, and Kinga Zapert. 2003. Common concerns amidst diverse systems: Health care experiences in five countries. *Health Affairs* 22, 3 (May/June): 106–18.

Blendon, Robert J., et al. 2001. Inequities in health care: A five country study. *Health Affairs* 21, 3 (May/June): 182–204.

Boase, Joan Price. 1996. Health reform or health care rationing? A comparative study. *Canadian–American Public Policy* 26 (May): 1–48.

———. 2001. Federalism and the health facility fee challenge. In *Federalism, democratic, and health policy in Canada,* ed. Duane Adams, 179–206. Montreal and Kingston: McGill-Queen's University Press.

Boychuk, Gerard W. 2002a. The changing political and economic environment of health care in Canada. Discussion Paper No. 1, Commission on the Future of Health Care in Canada, July 2002.

———. 2002b. Public health-care provision in the Canadian provinces and American states. *Canadian Public Administration* 45, 2 (Summer): 217–38.

———. 2002c. Federal spending in health . . . Why here? Why now? In *How Ottawa spends 2002–2003: The security aftermath and national priorities,* ed. G. Bruce Doern, 121–36. Don Mills: Oxford University Press.

———. 2003. The federal role in health care reform: Legacy or limbo? In *How Ottawa spends 2003–2004: The legacy agenda,* ed. G. Bruce Doern, 89–103. Don Mills: Oxford University Press.

———. 2004. The Chrétien non-legacy: The federal role in health care ten years on, 1993–2003. *Review of Constitutional Studies* (February 2004).

———. 2007. Patience! . . . Wait time guarantees: Harper and health care. In *How Ottawa spends, 2007/8,* eds. Bruce G. Doern. Kingston and Montréal: McGill-Queen's University Press.

———. 2008. Race, territorial integration and public policy in the United States and Canada. In *Canada and the United States: Differences that count, 3rd ed.,* eds. David M. Thomas and Barbara Torrey. Peterborough, ON: Broadview.

Boychuk, Gerard W., and Keith G. Banting, 2008. The private/public divide: Pensions and health insurance in Canada. In *Comparative social policy and the public–private dichotomy,* eds. Daniel Béland and Brian Gran. Houndmills, UK: Palgrave Macmillan.

British Columbia, Elections BC. 2005. *Electoral history of British Columbia, 1871–1986.* Available at www.elections.bc.ca/elections/electoral_history/toc.html.

Brown, Michael K. 1999. *Race, money, and the American welfare state*. Ithaca: Cornell University Press.

Byrd, W. Michael, and Linda A. Clayton. 2000. *An American health dilemma, vol. 1: A medical history of African Americans and the problem of race: Beginnings to 1900*. New York: Routledge.

———. 2002. *An American health dilemma, vol. 2: Race, medicine, and health care in the United States, 1900–2000*. New York: Routledge.

Canada. Department of Finance. 1999. *Strengthening health care for Canadians*. Ottawa: Finance Canada.

Canada. Department of Foreign Affairs and International Trade. 1996. Canada's health care system protected under the NAFTA. Available at http://webapps.dfait-maeci.gc.ca/min pub/Publication.asp?publication_id = 376 523&Language = E. Accessed on April 20, 2005.

Canada. First Ministers' Meeting. 1999. *A framework to improve the social union for Canadians*. First Ministers' Meeting, Ottawa, February.

Canada, Office of the Prime Minister. 2004b. "Asymmetrical Federalism that Respect's Quebec's Jurisdiction," http://pm.gc.ca/grfx/docs/QuebecENG.pdf.

Canadian Institute for Health Information. 2004. *Drug expenditure in Canada, 1985–2004*. Ottawa: Canadian Institute for Health Information.

Canadian Medical Association Journal. 1936. News Items. *Canadian Medical Association Journal* (February): 232.

CBC News Online. 2004. Wait times priority, not drugs, says health minister. *CBC News Online*, August 16.

CBS News, New York Times. 1991. August. Accessed from Roper Center for Public Opinion Research online via LexisNexis. [Accession Number: 0163304]

CIHI. *See* Canadian Institute Health Information.

Clark, Campbell. 2004. Health care key to Martin's plan. *Globe and Mail*, April 28.

Clinton, William J. 1994. *President Clinton's address before a joint session of the Congress on the State of the Union*. www.c-span.org/executive/transcript.asp?cat = current_event& code = bush_ad min&year = 1994. Accessed February 4, 2008.

Cobb, W. Montague. 1953. NAACP's resolutions on health. *Journal of the National Medical Association* 45: 438–39.

———. 1957. Integration in medicine: A national need. *Journal of the National Medical Association* 49, 1 (January): 1–7.

Cohen, Wilbur J. 1986. Reflections on the enactment of Medicare and Medicaid. *Health Care Financing Review*, Annual Supplement, 2–11.

———. 1986. Random reflections on the Great Society's politics and health care programs after twenty years. In *The Great Society and its legacy: Twenty years of US social policy*, ed. Marshall Kaplan and Peggy L. Cuciti, 113–20. Durham: Duke University Press.

Commission on Presidential Debates. 2004. *Debate transcript 2004*. Washington, DC: Commission on Presidential Debates. Available at www.debates.org/pages/trans2004a.html. Accessed February 12, 2008.

Commonwealth Fund. 2004. *2004 Commonwealth Fund international health policy survey of adults' experiences with primary care*. New York: Commonwealth Fund. Available at www.commonwealthfund.org/surveys/surveys_show.htm?doc_id = 245240.   Accessed February 5, 2008.

Congressional Record. 1945. 79th Cong., 1st Session. Vol. 91.

Congressional Record. 1947. 80th Cong., 1st Session. Vol. 93.

Congressional Record. 1948. 80th Cong., 2nd Session. Vol. 94.

Congressional Record. 1949. 81st Cong., 1st Session. Vol. 95.

Congressional Record. 1950. 81st Cong, 2nd Session. Vol. 96.

Congressional Record. 1951. 82nd Cong., 1st Session. Vol. 97.

Congressional Record. 1962. 87th Cong., 2nd Session. Vol. 97.

CCF. *See* Cooperative Commonwealth Federation.

Cooperative Commonwealth Federation. 1933. *Regina Manifesto.* Regina: CCF. Available at www.prairiecentre.com/manifesto.htm. Accessed February 23, 2005.

Cornely, Paul B. 1957. Trend in racial integration in hospitals in the United States. *Journal of the National Medical Association* 49, 1 (January): 8–10.

Corry, J. A. 1939. *Difficulties of divided jurisdiction: A study prepared for the Royal Commission on Dominion–Provincial Relations.* Ottawa: King's Printer.

Coughlin, Richard. 1980. *Ideology, public opinion and welfare policy: Attitudes towards taxes and spending in industrialized countries.* Berkeley: Institute of International Studies, University of California.

Council of the Federation. 2004. Premier's action plan for better health care: Resolving issues in the spirit of true federalism. Communiqué, July 30. Available at www.councilofthefederation.ca/pdfs/HealthEng.pdf.

Coyne, Andrew. 2004. What if Meech had a son? *National Post,* September 17, 1.

Curry, Bill. 2004. No one will mention private care: Layton, "elephant in the room." *National Post,* September 14, A5.

David, Alvin. 1966. Former Social Security Administration, Programming Planning official, interview transcript, Oral History Research Office, Columbia University. Available at www.ssa.gov/history/adavid66.html.

David, Sheri I. 1985. *With dignity: The search for Medicare and Medicaid.* Westport, CT: Greenwood Press.

Dawson, Anne. 2004. Québec deal health for federalism: PM. *National Post,* September 24, A1.

Detroit Free Press. 1949. Why we face state medicine—AMA rebuffs the progressive doctors. *Detroit Free Press,* February 28 (reprinted in *Congressional Record,* 1949: A1197).

Esmail, Nadeem, and Michael Walker. 2004. *Waiting your turn: Hospital waiting lists in Canada, 14th ed.* Vancouver: Fraser Institute.

Evans, Robert G. 2000. Two systems in restraint: Contrasting experiences with cost control in the 1900s. In *Canada and the United States: Differences that count, 2nd ed.,* ed. David M. Thomas, 21–51. Peterborough, ON: Broadview.

Ewing, Oscar R. 1948. *The nation's health: A report to the president.* Washington, DC: Federal Security Agency, 53, 35.

Families USA and Health Insurance Association of America. 1999. *Uninsured Americans survey.* October 12. Accessed from Roper Center for Public Opinion Research online via LexisNexis. [Accession Number: 0345081; Question 24, Accession Number 0345085; Question 22, Accession 03455083]

Fleeson, Doris. 1949. Powerful medicine: Coalition fight on Ewing imperils plan to combine welfare activities. *Washington Evening Star,* August 11. Reprinted in *Congressional Record,* 11445.

Flood, Colleen. 2002. Presentation to Ontario Health Coalition Public Form, Does Medicare Work? Toronto, April 3.

Fox, Daniel M., and John K. Inglehart. 1995. *Five states that could not wait: Lessons for health reform from Florida, Hawaii, Minnesota, Oregon and Vermont.* Cambridge, MA: Health Affairs and Milbank Memorial Fund.

Gilens, Martin. 1995. Racial attitudes and opposition to welfare. *Journal of Politics* 57, 4 (November): 994–1014.

———. 1999. *Why Americans hate welfare: Race, media and the politics of antipoverty policy.* Chicago: University of Chicago Press.

Goldfarb, Martin. 2004. Pharmacare: A tonic for federalism. *Globe and Mail*, September 7, A17.

Gordon, Walter L. 1977. *A political memoir.* Toronto: McClelland and Stewart.

Gottschalk, Marie. 2000. *The shadow welfare states: Labor, business, and the politics of health care in the United States.* Ithaca: ILR Press.

Granatstein, J. L. 1969. *Conscription in the Second World War, 1939–1945.* Toronto: Ryerson.

Grauer, A. E. 1939. *Public assistance and social insurance: A study prepared for the Royal Commission on Dominion–Provincial Relations.* Ottawa: King's Printer.

Grogan, Colleen. 1995. Hope in federalism? What can the states do and what are they likely to do? *Journal of Health Politics, Policy and Law* 20, 2 (Summer): 477–84.

———. 2007. A marriage of convenience: The history of nursing home coverage and Medicaid. In *Putting the past back in: History and health policy in the United States,* ed. R. A. Stevens, C. E. Rosenberg, and L. R. Burns. New Brunswick, NJ: Rutgers University Press.

Grogan, C. M., and Patashnik, E. 2003a. Between welfare medicine and mainstream program: Medicaid at the political crossroads. *Journal of Health Politics, Policy and Law* 28, 5 (October): 821–58.

———. 2003b. Universalism within targeting: Nursing home care, the middle class, and the politics of the Medicaid Program. *Social Service Review* 77(1): 51–71.

Guest, Dennis. 1997. *The emergence of social security in Canada, 3rd ed.* Vancouver: University of British Columbia Press.

Hacker, Jacob S. 1997. *The road to nowhere: The genesis of President Clinton's plan for health security.* Princeton, NJ: Princeton University Press.

———. 1998. The historical logic of national health insurance: Structure and development of British, Canadian, and U.S. Medical Policy. *Studies in American Political Development* 12 (Spring): 57–130.

———. 2002. *The divided welfare state: The battle over public and private social benefits in the United States.* Cambridge: Cambridge University Press.

———. 2004. Privatizing risk without privatizing the welfare state: The hidden politics of social policy retrenchment in the United States. *American Political Science Review* 98, 2 (May): 243–60.

Harris, Richard. 1966. *A sacred trust.* New York: New American Library.

Harvard School of Public Health and Kaiser Family Foundation. 1994. *Health reform project survey—Wave 2.* February. Accessed from Roper Center for Public Opinion Research online via LexisNexis. [Accession Number: 0231596]

Harvard School of Public Health and Robert Wood Johnson Foundation. 2001. *Health insurance coverage survey.* September 10. Accessed from Roper Center for Public Opinion Research online via LexisNexis. [Accession Number: 0389881; Question 14, Accession Number 0389846]

Harvard University and Kaiser Family Foundation. 1995. *Washington Post/Harvard/Kaiser Family Foundation race relations poll.* December 1. Accessed from Roper Center for Public Opinion Research online via LexisNexis. [Accession Number: 255622]

Harvey, Lynn K. 1993. *Public opinion on health care issues.* Chicago: American Medical Association.

Haseltine, N. S. 1949. AMA imposes gag on Dr. Fishbein. *Washington Post*, June 7, 2.

Health Canada. 2000. Health minister launches Canadian Institutes of Health Research. News release, June 7. Available at www.hc-sc.gc.ca/english/archives/releases/2000/cihre.htm.

———. 2003. First ministers agree on 2003 first ministers' accord on health care renewal. www.hc-sc.gc.ca/english/hca2003/accord.html. Accessed May 30, 2005.

———. 2004. *The 2003 accord on health care renewal: A progress report.* Available at www .hc-sc.gc.ca/english/media/releases/2004/fmm01.htm. Accessed on May 30, 2005.

Health Care in Canada. 2001. *Health care in Canada survey 2001: A national survey of health care providers, managers and the public.* Available at www.mediresource.com/e/pages/ hcc_survey/pdf/2001_hcic.pdf.

Hess, Arthur E. 1996. Interview with Arthur Hess, former director of health insurance for Medicare, 1965–67. Health Care Financing Agency Collection. July.

Houston, C. Stuart. 2002. *Steps on the road to Medicare: Why Saskatchewan led the way?* Montreal and Kingston: McGill-Queen's University Press.

Huber, Manfred, and Eva Orosz. 2003. Health expenditure trends in OECD countries, 1990–2001. *Health Care Financing Review* 25, 1 (Fall): 1–23.

Hutchings, Vincent L. and Nicholas A. Valentino. 2004. "The Centrality of Race in American Politics" *Annual Review of Political Science* 7 (2004): 383–408.

Inglehart, John K. 1999a. The American health care system: Expenditures. *New England Journal of Medicine* 340, 1 (January 7): 72.

———. 1999b. The American health care system: Medicare. *New England Journal of Medicine* 340, 4 (January 28): 328.

———. 1999c. The American health care system: Medicaid. *New England Journal of Medicine* 340, 5 (February 4): 403, 407, 403.

Ipsos-Reid. 2005. A public opinion survey of Canadians and Americans: Report prepared for the Canada Institute of the Woodrow Wilson International Center and the Canadian Institute on North American Issues. Toronto: Ipsos-Reid.

Iton, Richard. 2000. *Solidarity blues: Race, culture, and the American left.* Chapel Hill: University of North Carolina Press.

JNMA. *See Journal of the National Medical Association.*

Jones, James H. 1993. *Bad blood: The Tuskegee syphilis experiment.* New York: Free Press.

Journal of the American Medical Association. 1949. The president's message and the compulsory health insurance bill. *Journal of the American Medical Association* 140, 1 (May 7): 111–12.

Journal of the National Medical Association. 1960. Elimination of racial discrimination in hospital practices. *Journal of the National Medical Association* 52, 3 (May): 199–200.

———. 1962a. Dingell bill to end hospital discrimination under the Hill–Burton Act. *Journal of the National Medical Association* (May): 388–89.

———. 1962b. Green bill to end hospital discrimination under the Hill–Burton Act. *Journal of the National Medical Association* (September): 628–29.

———. 1962c. Hospital discrimination and the sixth Imhotep conference. *Journal of the National Medical Association* (March): 253–59.

Kaiser Family Foundation. 1999. *Race, ethnicity, and medical care survey.* October. Accessed from Roper Center for Public Opinion Research online via LexisNexis. [Accession Number: 0341971]

———. 2004. *Health poll report.* April 15. Accessed from Roper Center for Public Opinion Research online via LexisNexis. [Accession Number: 451709]

Kaiser Family Foundation and Harvard School of Public Health. 1993. *Public knowledge of health reform survey.* October. Accessed from Roper Center for Public Opinion Research online via LexisNexis. [Accession Number: 0409019]

Katznelson, Ira. 2005. *When affirmative action was white: An untold history of racial inequality in twentieth-century America.* New York: Norton.

King, Desmond. 1995. *Separate and unequal: Black Americans and the US federal government.* Oxford: Oxford University Press.

Kingdon, John W. 1984. *Agendas, alternatives, and public policies.* Boston: Little Brown.

Klarman, Michael J. 1994. How *Brown* changed race relations: The backlash thesis. *Journal of American History* 81, 1 (June): 81–118.

Knowless, Clayton. 1949. First Truman plan in reorganization beaten in Senate: Debate centers on Ewing. *New York Times,* August 17, 1.

Kudrle, Robert T., and Theodore R. Marmor. 1981. The development of welfare states in North America. In *The development of welfare states in Europe and North America,* ed. Peter Flora and Arnold J. Heidenheimer, 81–121. New Brunswick: Transaction.

La Marsh, Judy. 1969. *Memoirs of a bird in a gilded cage.* Toronto: McClelland and Stewart.

Lambton, John George. 1839. *Report on the affairs of British North America* [*The Durham Report*]. Accessed at http://faculty.marianopolis.edu/c.belanger/quebechistory/docs/durham/.

Laurence, William. 1949a. AMA glosses over the Fishbein case. *New York Times,* June 8, 31–32.

———. 1949b. AMA to retire Dr. Fishbein after he trains new editors. *New York Times,* June 7, 1–2.

Liberal Party of Canada. 1993. *Creating opportunity: The Liberal plan for Canada.* Ottawa: Liberal Party of Canada.

———. 1997. *Securing our future together: Preparing Canada for the 21st century.* Ottawa: Liberal Party of Canada.

———. 2000. *Opportunity for all: The Liberal plan for the future of Canada.* Ottawa: Liberal Party of Canada.

———. 2004. Strengthening our social foundations. Ottawa: Liberal Party of Canada. www.liberal.ca/platform_e_3.aspx.

Lieberman, Robert C. 1998. *Shifting the color line: Race and the American welfare state.* Cambridge, MA: Harvard University Press.

Lipset, Seymour Martin. 1990. *Continental divide: The values and institutions of the United States and Canada.* New York: Routledge.

Magner, W. 1949. Health insurance. *Canadian Medical Association Journal* 61 (August): 184–87.

Maioni, Antonia. 1998. *Parting at the crossroads: The emergence of health insurance in the United States and Canada.* Princeton, NJ: Princeton University Press.

———. 2002. The citizenship-building effects of Canada's universal health care regime. *Revista Mexicana de Estudios Canadienses* 5 (Winter 2002). Available at http://revista.amec.com.mx/num_5_2002/Maioni_Antonia.htm. Accessed on February 4, 2008.

Marmor, Theodore R. 1970. *The politics of Medicare.* Chicago: Aldine.

———. 1994. *Understanding health care reform.* New Haven: Yale University Press.

———. 2000. *The politics of Medicare. 2nd ed.* New York: Aldine.

Marmor, T., K. Okma, and S. Latham, 2002. *National values, institutions and health policy: What do they imply for medicare reform?* Ottawa: Royal Commission on the Future of Health Care in Canada.

Mayes, Rick. 2004a. Universal coverage, health inequalities, and the American health care system in crisis (again). *Journal of Health Care Law and Policy* 7, 2.

———. 2004b. *Universal coverage: The elusive question for national health insurance.* Ann Arbor: University of Michigan Press.

McCoy, Donald R., and Richard R. Ruetten. 1973. *Quest and response: Minority rights and the Truman administration.* Lawrence: University Press of Kansas.

McCullough, David. 1992. *Truman.* New York: Simon and Schuster.

McDaniel, R. 1985. Management and medicine: Never the twain shall meet. *Journal of the National Medical Association* 77, 2: 107–12.

McDougall, Barbara. 2001. Free trade: Ten years on. Address to the Canadian Pension & Benefits Institution and the International Foundation of Employee Benefits Plans Conference, June 21. Available at www.ciia.org/speech7.htm. Accessed on April 20, 2005.

Mendelsohn, Matthew. 2001. *Canadians' thoughts on their health care system: Preserving the Canadian model through innovation.* Ottawa: Royal Commission on the Future of Health Care in Canada.

Meyer, Agnes E. 1949. Social legislation in the 81st Congress. *Washington Post*, January 20, C6.

Mink, Gwendolyn. 1995. *The wages of motherhood: Inequality and the welfare state, 1917–1942.* Ithaca: Cornell University Press.

———. 1998. *Welfare's end.* Ithaca: Cornell University Press.

Mitchell, Daniel J. B. 2002. Impeding Earl Warren: California's health insurance plan that wasn't and what might have been. California: UCLA Human Resources Round Table Working Paper, March. Available at www.harrt.ucla.edu/publications/workingpapers/Mitchell.pdf.

Morais, Herbert M. 1967. *The history of the Negro in medicine.* New York: Publishers Company.

Morone, James. 1990. *The Democratic wish: Popular participation and the limits of American government.* New York: Basic Books.

———. 1995. Nativism, hollow corporations, and managed competition: Why the Clinton health care reform failed. *Journal of Health Politics, Policy and Law* 20, 2 (Summer): 391–98.

———. 2003. American ways of welfare. *Perspectives on Politics* 1, 1 (March): 137–46.

———. 2004. *Hellfire nation.* New Haven: Yale University Press.

Morris, John P. 1960. The denial of staff positions to Negro physicians: A violation of the Sherman Act. *Journal of the National Medical Association* 52, 3 (May): 211–12.

Murray, Charles. 1984. *Losing ground: American social policy, 1950–1980.* New York: Basic Books.

Myrdal, Gunnar. 1944. *An American dilemma: The Negro problem and modern democracy.* New York: Harper and Brothers.

NAACP. *See* National Association for the Advancement of Colored People.

National Academy of Social Insurance. 2001. Restructuring Medicare for the long term project, study panel on Medicare management and governance. *Reflections on Implementing Medicare.* Washington, DC: NASI.

National Association for the Advancement of Colored People. 1950. Race tag removed from blood. *The Crisis* (December): 714–15.

———. 1957a. New hospital group. *The Crisis* (April): 219–20.

———. 1957b. NAACP goals for 1963. *The Crisis* (April): 560–61.

———. Legal defense and education fund, 1989. *Unfinished agenda on race.* January 1989. Accessed from Roper Center for Public Opinion Research online via LexisNexis. [Accession Number: 0074247]

National Conference of Christians and Jews, Ford Foundation, and Joyce Foundation. 1994. *National conference survey on inter-group relations.* March 2. Accessed from Roper Center for Public Opinion Research online via LexisNexis. [Accession Number: 227164]

National Forum on Health. 1997. *Canada health action: Building on the legacy, vol. 4: Health care systems in Canada and elsewhere.* Sainte Foy, PQ: Éditions MultiMondes.

National Governors' Association. 2000. Health Policy Studies Division. *ERISA case law update*, May. Available at www.nga.org/pubs/issueBriefs/2000/000501ERISA.pdf.

Naylor, David C. 1986. *Private practice, public payment: Canadian medicine and the politics of health insurance, 1911–1966.* Kingston and Montreal: McGill-Queen's University Press.

Newman, Peter C. 1968. *The distemper of our times: Canadian politics in transition, 1963–1968.* Toronto: McClelland and Stewart.

New York Times. 1948. Anti-bias move in AMA demanded. March 23, 29.

———. 1949a. AMA choice of Negro is called 'political.' August 12, 10.

———. 1949b. Doctors defeated, FSA head asserts. December 15, 37.

———. 1949c. Doctor group backs Truman health plans. June 23, 31.

———. 1949d. Doctors of county shift on AMA Levy. March 1, 27.

———. 1949e. Fight health plan, AMA Asks Negroes. August 10, 18.

———. 1949f. GOP health plan assailed by Ewing. June 2, 18.

———. 1949g. Negro doctors defer health plan. August 13.

———. 1949h. Negro seen denied even skimpy care. June 28, 29.

———. 1949i. Proposed national FEPC bill arouses strong sentiment. May 15, E7.

———. 1949j. Race bias denied by medical group. March 2.

———. 1957. AMA president scores plan to give health benefits to aged. December 4, 32.

———. 1964a. Still blocking Medicare. May 26, 38.

———. 1964b. One-man veto on Medicare. June 26, 28.

———. 1964c. Movement on Medicare? November 13, 34.

———. 1965a. Medicare moves into law. July 29, 26.

———. 1965b. New AMA chief warns against medicare boycott. June 21, 1.

———. 1965c. AMA chiefs ask delay on boycott. June 24, 46.

———. 1965d. Doctors' group says AMA aids 'evil' by Medicare stand. August 14, 20.

———. 1965e. Medicare drive on rights urged. December 17, 2.

Nichols, Len M., and Linda J. Blumberg. 1998. A different kind of 'New Federalism'? The Health Insurance Portability and Accountability Act of 1996. *Health Affairs* 17, 3 (May/June): 25–42.

NYT. *See New York Times.*

Oberlander, Jonathan. 2003. *The political life of Medicare.* Chicago: University of Chicago Press.

OECD. *See* Organization for Economic Cooperation and Development.

Organization for Economic Cooperation and Development. 2006. *OECD health data 2006* [CD-ROM]. Paris: OECD.

Orren, Karen, and Stephen Skowronek. 2004. *The search for American political development.* Cambridge, UK: Cambridge University Press.

Pear, Robert. 2007. Senate passes children's health bill, 68–31. *New York Times,* August 3, online edition.

Pierson, Paul and Theda Skocpol. 2002. "Historical Institutionalism in Contemporary Political Science," 693–721 in Ira Katznelson and Helen V. Milner, ed., *Political Science: State of the Discipline.* New York: Norton.

Pierson, Paul. 2004. *Politics in time: History, institutions and social analysis.* Princeton, NJ: Princeton University Press.

Pipes, Shelley. 2004. *Miracle cure: How to solve America's health care crisis and why Canada isn't the answer.* San Francisco: Pacific Research Institute.

Poen, Monte S. 1979. *Harry S. Truman versus the medical lobby: The genesis of Medicare.* Columbia: University of Missouri Press.

Polsky, Allyson D. 2002. Blood, race and national identity: Scientific and popular discourses. *Journal of Medical Humanities*, 23, 3/4 (Winter): 171–86.

Porter, John. 1965. *The Vertical Mosaic: An Analysis of Social Class and Power in Canada.* Toronto: University of Toronto Press.

Quadagno, Jill S. 1988. *Transformation of old age security: Class and politics in the American welfare state.* Chicago: University of Chicago Press.

———. 1994. *The color of welfare: How racism undermined the war on poverty.* New York: Oxford University Press.

———. 2005. *One nation uninsured: Why the U.S. has no national health insurance.* New York: Oxford University Press.

Raffel, Margaret A., Marshall W. Raffel, and Norma K. Raffel. 1997. The health system of the United States. In *Health care and reform in industrialized countries,* ed. Marshall W. Raffel, 263–89. University Park: Pennsylvania State University Press.

Reynolds, P. Preston. 1997b. "Hospitals and Civil Rights, 1945–1963: The Case of Simkins v. Moses H. Cone Memorial Hospital." *Annals of Internal Medicine.* 126, 11 (June): 898–906.

———. 1997b. Hospitals and civil rights, 1945–1963: The case of Simkins *v.* Moses H. Cone Memorial Hospital. *Annals of Internal Medicine* 126, 11 (June): 898–906.

Robert Wood Johnson Foundation and Harvard School of Public Health. 1993. *American attitudes toward health care reform.* May 16. Accessed from Roper Center for Public Opinion Research online via LexisNexis. [Accession Number: 0197044]

Rom, Mark C. 1999. Transforming state health and welfare programs. In *Politics in the American states: A comparative analysis, 7th ed.,* 351. Washington, DC: Congressional Quarterly.

Romanow, Roy J. 2002. *Building on values: The future of health care in Canada, final report.* Ottawa: Commission on the Future of Health Care in Canada, xi.

Rorem, C. Rufus. 1931. *The "municipal doctor" system in rural Saskatchewan.* Publications of the Committee on the Costs of Medical Care, No. 11. Chicago: University of Chicago Press.

Royal Commission on Dominion–Provincial Relations. 1939. *Report of the Royal Commission on Dominion–Provincial Relations, book II – recommendations.* Ottawa: Queen's Printer.

Schiltz, Michael E. 1970. *Public attitudes toward social security, 1935–1965.* Washington, DC: U.S. Department of Health, Education and Welfare, Social Security Administration, Office of Research and Statistics.

Schlesinger, Mark, and Taeku Lee. 1994. Is health care different? Popular support of federal health and social policies. In *The politics of health care reform: Lessons from the past, prospects for the future,* ed. James A. Morone and Gary S. Belkin, 297–374. Durham: Duke University Press.

Shearon, Marjorie. 1940. A review of state legislation relating to medical services and to cash payments for disability, proposed during 1939. *Social Security Bulletin* (January): 34–51.

Skocpol, Theda. 1992. *Protecting soldiers and mothers: The political origins of social policy in the United States.* Cambridge, MA: Belknap Press.

———. 1996. *Boomerang: Health care reform and the turn against government.* New York: Norton.

Smith, David Barton. 1999. *Health care divided: Race and healing a nation.* Ann Arbor: University of Michigan Press.

———. 2005. *Eliminating disparities in treatment and the struggle to end segregation.* Commonwealth Fund Publication No. 775. New York: Commonwealth Fund.

Sokoloff, Heather. 2004. A province of private clinics. *National Post,* September 9, A1.

Somers, Herman Miles and Anne Ramsay Somers. *Doctors, Patients, and Health Insurance: The Organization and Financing of Medical Care.* Washington: Brookings Institution, 1961.

Sparer, Michael S. 1994. The unknown states. In *The politics of health care reform: Lessons from the past, prospects for the future,* ed. James A. Morone and Gary S. Belkin, 430–39. Durham and London: Duke University Press.

Spargo, Mary. 1949. 23 Democrats join GOP block of 37 in rejection despite White House appeal. *Washington Post,* August 17, 1.

Stanbury, W. T. 1996. Cancon rules should be canned. *Policy Options* 17, 9 (October): 25–28.

Starr, Paul. 1982. *The social transformation of American medicine.* New York: Basic Books.

Statistics Canada. 2004. Available at www.statcan.ca/.

Steinmo, Sven, and Jon Watts. 1995. It's the institutions, stupid! Why comprehensive national health insurance always fails in America. *Journal of Health Politics, Policy and Law* 20, 2 (Summer): 329–72.

Strunk, Mildred. 1946. The quarter's polls. *Public Opinion Quarterly* 10, 4 (Winter 1946–47): 623.

———. 1949. The quarter's polls. *Public Opinion Quarterly* 13, 1 (Spring).

Stucke, Adela. 1952. Notes on compulsory sickness insurance legislation in the states, 1939–44. *Public Health Reports* 60, 52 (December 28): 1551–64.

Sundquist, James L. 1968. *Politics and policy: The Eisenhower, Kennedy, and Johnson years.* Washington, DC: Brookings Institution.

Taylor, Malcolm G. 1954. Social assistance medical care programs in Canada. *American Journal of Public Health,* 44 (June): 750–59.

———. 1987. *Health insurance and Canadian public policy: The seven decisions that created the Canadian health insurance system and their outcomes,* 2d ed. Kingston and Montreal: McGill-Queen's University Press.

———. 1990. *Insuring national health care: The Canadian experience.* Chapel Hill: University of North Carolina Press.

Terry, Luther L. 1965. "Hospitals and Title VI of the Civil Rights Act." *Hospitals—The Journal of the American Hospital Association* 39, 1 (August):34–7.

Thelen, Kathleen. 2003. How institutions evolve: Insights from comparative historical analysis. In *Comparative historical analysis in the social sciences,* ed. James Mahoney and Dietrich Rueschemeyer, 208–40. Cambridge: Cambridge University Press.

Thompson, Dorothy. 1948. On the record. *New York Mirror,* December 26. 1948. Reprinted in *Congressional Record,* A225.

Thorpe, Kenneth E. 1994. American states and Canadian provinces: A comparative analysis of health care spending. In *The politics of health care reform: Lessons from the past, prospects for the future,* ed. James A. Morone and Gary S. Belkin, 405–17. Durham: Duke University Press, 1994.

Titmuss, Richard M. 1970. *The gift relationship: From human blood to social policy.* London: George Allen and Unwin.

Toner, Robin. 2003. An imperfect compromise. *New York Times,* November, A1

Truman, Harry S. 1947. Address to the NAACP. June 28. Available at www.pbs.org/wgbh/amex/truman/psources/ps_naacp.html.

Tuohy, Carolyn Hughes. 1999. *Accidental logics: The dynamics of change in the health care arena in the United States, Britain and Canada.* New York: Oxford University Press.

U.S. Senate. Committee on Expenditures in the Executive Departments. 1949. *Hearings on reorganization plans no. 1 and no. 2 of 1949.* Washington, DC: GPO.

U.S. Senate. Committee on Finance. 1970. *Medicare and Medicaid: Problems, issues and alternatives.* Washington, DC: GPO.

U.S. Senate. Committee on Labor and Public Welfare. Subcommittee on Health. 1947. *National health program: Hearings on S. 545 and S. 1320, part 1.* Washington, DC: GPO.

————. Subcommittee on Health Legislation. 1949. *National health program, 1949—part 1.* Washington, DC: GPO.

————. Subcommittee on Hospital Construction and Local Public Health Units. 1949. *Hospital survey and construction (Hill–Burton) act amendments.* Washington, DC: GPO.

Vaillancourt-Rosenau, Pauline. 1992. National health insurance in the United States and Canada: The role of political structure and process. Paper delivered to the Annual Meeting of the American Political Science Association.

Vallières, Pierre. 1970. *White niggers of America.* Toronto: McClelland and Stewart.

Vladeck, Bruce C. 1980. *Unloving care: The nursing home tragedy.* New York: Basic Books.

Washington Post, Kaiser Family Foundation, and Harvard University. 2000. *Washington Post, Kaiser, Harvard 2000 election health care survey.* July 28. Accessed from Roper Center for Public Opinion Research online via LexisNexis. [Accession Number: 0427726]

Williams, Linda F. 2003. *The constraint of race: Legacies of white skin privilege in America.* University Park: Pennsylvania State University Press.

Wing, Kenneth R., and Marilyn G. Rose. 1980. Health facilities and the enforcement of civil rights. In *Legal aspects of health policy: Issues and trends,* ed. Ruther Roemer and George McKray, 243–67. Westport, CT: Greenwood.

Witte, Edwin E. 1963. *The development of the Social Security Act.* Madison: University of Wisconsin Press.

Woolhandler S., T. Campbell, and D. U. Himmelstein. 2003. Costs of health care administration in the United States and Canada. *New England Journal of Medicine* 349: 768–75.

Zelizer, Julian E. 1998. *Taxing America: Wilbur D. Mills, Congress, and the state, 1945–1975.* Cambridge: Cambridge University Press.

INDEX

Note: Page numbers followed by "t" or "f" indicate tables and figures in the text.

access to health care (contemporary U.S./Canada comparisons), 177–80, 180f
Aid to Dependent Children (ADC), 24, 69
Aid to Families with Dependent Children (AFDC), 75, 89, 199n22
Alberta: alternative universal public insurance proposal (1960s), 128; CHA and extra-billing issue, 139; early public health insurance initiatives, 36–37; and federal deal of 2004, 151; municipal hospital care plan (1950), 203n15; public preferences regarding private delivery of health services, 152
Altmeyer, Arthur, 29
American Association for Labor Legislation (AALL), 27, 32
American exceptionalism, 3, 4–5, 92, 140
American Medical Association (AMA): and CMA, 32, 101; critics of, 55–56; history of forestalling reform/opposition to reforms, 192; internal dissent, 54; Medicare opposition campaign, 63, 71, 121, 198n4, 199nn17–18; members' financial dues, 121; organizational structure and the segregated medical profession, 25, 47, 49, 197n4; Truman-era campaign against national compulsory health insurance, 46, 47, 49, 50, 53–56
American Red Cross and blood segregation policy, 26
Anderson, Clinton, 63, 198n4

Ball, Robert M., 57, 61, 66–67, 73
Banting, Keith G., 9, 162
Barer, Morris C., 157
Bégin, Monique, 138
Bennett, R. B., 34
Bertrand, Jean-Jacques, 207n27
Blendon, Robert J., 88, 91, 211n25
Blue, Rupert, 22
Borden, Robert, 33
British Columbia: alternative universal public insurance proposal (1960s), 128, 206n5; early initiative (1919), 35; hospital insurance, 106; postwar hospital insurance and administrative problems, 106; postwar reforms, 102–3, 106; public health insurance reform (1930s), 34–37, 197n15; public preferences regarding private delivery of health services, 152
British Columbia College of Physicians and Surgeons, 35
British Columbia Medical Association (BCMA), 36, 101
British Columbia Medical Plan (BCMP), 206n5
British North America Act, 13–14, 32, 202–3n9
Broadbent, Ed, 137
Brown decision (1954), 29, 60–62, 64
Bush, George W., 3, 171
Byrd, Harry, 66

California Medical Association, 30, 121
California public health insurance initiatives (1910–45), 26, 30–31, 34, 196nn8–9; Progressive-Era ballot initiative (1918), 26; Warren Plan, 30–31, 196n9
Campbell, T., 181
Canada and contemporary public health insurance: access to health care, 177–80, 180f; access to specialists and surgical care, 176–77, 182–83; administrative costs, 181; comparing coverage and provision with American states, 162–70; comparing with U.S. system/states, 158–70; coverage, 163–64, 210n10; doctor choice, 168–69; effectiveness, 174–75, 175t; emergency waiting times, 176; expenditures on hospitals and physicians, 209n2; hospital funding, 170; medical inflation/price indices for total medical expenditures, 182, 182t; out-of-pocket costs/expenditures, 179, 179t; performance assessments, 170–83; physicians' perceptions of performance, 172, 177–79; primary care (timeliness of access to), 176; the private-public mix and expenditures, 164–66; provinces' proscriptions on private third-party insurance, 159; provincial differences in coverage/expenditures, 166; provision of health services, 168–70; public